Badass and Bendy

A Yogi's Breast Cancer Story

Cathleen Kahn

Illustrator, Julie Coyle

BALBOA.
PRESS
A DIVISION OF HAY HOUSE

Balboa Press books may be ordered through booksellers or by contacting:

Balboa Press
A Division of Hay House
1663 Liberty Drive
Bloomington, IN 47403
www.balboapress.com
1 (877) 407-4847

Print information available on the last page.

ISBN: 978-1-9822-1630-6 (sc)
ISBN: 978-1-9822-1632-0 (hc)
ISBN: 978-1-9822-1631-3 (e)

Library of Congress Control Number: 2018913650

Balboa Press rev. date: 11/29/2018

Contents

Yoga Flows

Yoga Poses

Dedication

To
Edward, the love of my life, my laughter, and my heart. You
encouraged me, pushed me and made this a reality.
Samantha and Mackenzie, my children and my joy.
My family and friends who loved me through it.
Sandy, who read my words, told me I had to get
it out into the world and helped me edit.
Julie, who created the brilliant and whimsical
illustrations for the book.
All my West of the Moon Writers Retreat friends, I love the
support and enthusiasm I have always received from you.
To the yogi's I have taught and flowed with, you are my foundation.
To all those who have been affected by cancer, I hope this helps.

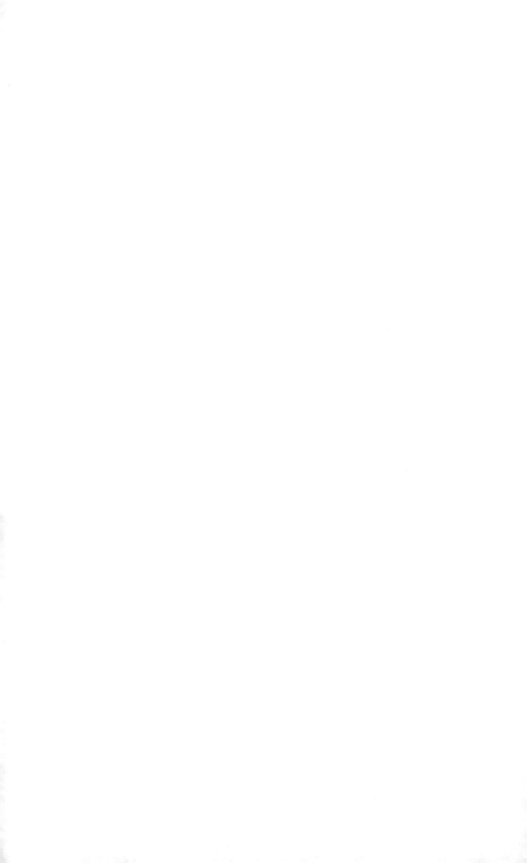

Introduction

I notice the world around me now. I notice the things that I imagine most people move right by and never see each day. I notice the color of the sky, not just that it is blue, but the different shades of blue. I see the leaves on the trees, each unique, individual leaf. I see how the sun catches the backs of the leaves and they look silver. I listen for the sounds of the different birds, the bark of a dog when I go on a walk, the way the wind blows over a mud puddle and makes it look magical. I am aware of the emotions on people's faces. I appreciate the sunrise, the sunset and each breath.

If you had asked me on November 12, 2006 if I noticed all the joy around me, I would've said of course. I thought I was aware. I thought I was happy. I didn't realize I was just existing as life happened around me.

On November 13, 2006 I was 45 years old.

Looking back at that woman, I see now what I couldn't see then.

I was a wife who made a loving home for my husband, David. I worked part-time yet made sure I was home before he was each day. I liked being a wife and fixing dinner. I loved to meet him at the door and welcome him home. I supported all of the PCS (permanent change of duty stations) moves he made as a military officer and I supported him as my husband. I was a military wife. I took the PCS moves, the trainings and the deployments in stride. That's what military spouses do. When you marry a soldier, you marry the military too.

I was a mother. I taught my children, Samantha and Mack, the importance of education. I gave them the love of books and curiosity. I taught them to have fun, to love life and to laugh. My children have never doubted that they were loved. They knew they were loved and accepted as they were.

I was a volunteer. I believed that "service is rent we pay for space on this planet". I have searched for the author of this quote and found credits to Muhammad Ali, Marian Wright Edelman, Shirley Chisholm and finally to an unknown inscription over a doorway in India in 1917. I do not know who said it first, but I believe it and I taught my children the importance of helping others.

I took pride in helping people improve their health. I began teaching fitness in 1987 while living at Schofield Barracks, Hawaii. I loved teaching everything from aerobics, to step aerobics, kickboxing, body sculpting classes, Taekwondo and yoga. I loved seeing the changes in the people I worked with. I worked hard to stay up-to-date on all of the latest research in the field of fitness. On November 12, 2006 – I was teaching eight classes a week and had five personal training clients a week.

I was all of those things, but I was also insecure, and I didn't know that I could be strong until I had to be strong. I had always had someone to take care of me. I knew that if anything bad was going to happen, someone else would be there to help me. I never had to depend on my strength. I was a strong woman when it came to my family, my friends and my work. I didn't know how to take care of *me*.

My life wasn't unique. I think many women could insert themselves into my story on November 12, 2006. On November 13, 2006, when I was told, "you have cancer," my known world was gone. I had to be strong.

Cancer changed me. The day I was diagnosed with cancer, there was no light at the end of the tunnel. There was only fear. Having to look my mortality in the face and acknowledge that I might die was like having an ice-cold bucket of water tossed on my naked body. On that day, there was only me, the numbing cold, and cancer.

Cancer took my belief that I would always be healthy. It forced me to look at the way I was living my life. I wanted more. I believe that I would still be married to David and just existing if I had not had cancer. I have been asked if cancer caused my divorce. It did not, but cancer made me aware of how unhappy I was. Four years after my divorce, I met a man, Edward, who loves me unconditionally. He doesn't try to change me. He loves me for who I am. That is the most remarkable gift I have ever received. I did not think that kind of love, acceptance and appreciation was real. I used to read historical romance novels and chuckle to myself at the absurdity of being loved completely. I thought it was a fairytale written for women like me who wanted to believe there was more.

Cancer gave my children a strong woman as their mother. They loved me completely before cancer. They believed I was intelligent, loving and full of life. I'm not sure that they believed I was strong until I battled cancer. Cancer took much from me but the changes in me would not have been possible without that experience. I wish I had been able to come to this end without having gone through cancer, but I would not change any part of my story. Cancer changed me, and fortunately, it didn't kill me. I was lucky.

One night over dinner with Edward, we were talking about awareness. I told him I believe we all notice the beauty and joy in life more as we age. I feel that the experiences that come with age can cause us to slow down and notice the world and the people around you. He disagreed with me. He felt that most people are less aware of their surroundings as they age. They stop looking at the world as new and exciting. Edward is a joyous, positive person so I was taken aback by his comment.

I think facing cancer makes you more sensitive to life. I see this awareness in my friend and yoga student Emily. She notices when someone is in need. She brings Chinese herbs in for yogis that have mentioned they have sore muscles. She sees a beautiful flower in her garden and brings it to the studio in a vase for all to enjoy. She is an incredible, giving soul. Emily, like me, had breast cancer. Once, I asked her after class if she felt she was more in tune with others and her surroundings now than she was before she had breast cancer. She said, "Absolutely. When you have something happen to you that causes you to face the fact you could die, you are different. You see things around you more."

Cancer gave me the strength to take charge of my life. We have all heard the cliché, "you only live once". We have paused to agree, then kept on living life as we had been living it. When you are given a diagnosis of cancer you have to face the fact that you do just have only one life to live.

If I had not had cancer, I do not believe I would have gone back to school and gotten my bachelor's or master's degree. Having those pieces of paper were important to me. I did not believe I could do it, but I did. I am not any smarter now than I was before I finished school, but those pieces of paper gave me confidence.

Yoga changed for me as well. Before cancer I saw yoga as just another fitness activity. During and after cancer it was a place of healing and acceptance. I got through cancer because of the strength of my children, my desire to stay strong for them and my yoga practice.

I told Edward that going through the diagnosis, the surgery, the treatment and the recovery would have been so much easier if I had been with him. He said, "Yes, it would have been, but you would not have become the person you are today."

I like the person I am today. I like her positivity, her strength and her desire to help others.

When I was going through chemotherapy, I tried to be positive and proactive. Did I cry? Oh yes, I cried. I cried because I was scared, I cried because I was mad at my body for betraying me and I cried because I was just plain tired. I did not let that change my belief that I would be healed, that I would get through this. My oncologist, Dr. Cobos, asked me to attend a support group for cancer patients. He said I could help them. I did not go. I have felt guilty about not going for years. I have wondered if I could have made a difference in someone's journey during that time. I did not have enough strength to share my story and my hope then.

I hope this book helps someone now.

Daddy's Warrior Princess

My daddy always called me Princess. I never wanted to be a warrior. My dad was a warrior, my brothers were warriors, my sister married a warrior and my ex-husband was a warrior. But, I became a warrior. I was diagnosed with breast cancer in November 2006. That diagnosis changed my life.

I am the firstborn of 6 children. My father was a military man. He was a General in the Army National Guard. He was a full-time Guardsman, so we were different from the regular army, but I was still an Army Brat. I married the army at age 23. My ex-husband was a regular army officer and an airborne ranger. The military was my way of life.

I am a mother of two children. Samantha is 26 years old. She is beautiful, intelligent, compassionate and strong. Mack is 22 years old. He is handsome, talented, loving and protective.

I am a yogi. I began teaching and working in the fitness industry at Schofield Barracks, Hawaii in 1987. Yoga was not a path I chose to follow. It was chosen for me. I was working as the Fitness Director and fitness instructor at a gym in Lubbock, Texas when we decided to add yoga to the schedule. I completed a yoga teacher training course. Yoga helped me to find who I am. Yoga was there for me at times when most of my strength was gone.

I am a learner. I love to learn. I got married when I was a senior in college and went back to school as an adult. I finished my bachelor's degree and completed a master's degree in business and a graduate certificate in creative writing.

I am a writer. It took me many years to consider myself a writer, but I write so I must be a writer.

There are many pieces that make me who I am.

Daddy's princess does not get cancer.

But I did.

Yoga Accepted Me

Every year in October I am reminded that I am a breast cancer survivor. The other 11 months of the year I pretend I am like everyone else but when September rolls around and I begin seeing all the pink ribbons in the stores, the memories and the fears resurface. It is at this time that I appreciate my yoga practice even more.

Before I was diagnosed with breast cancer in November 2006, yoga was a part of my life. I had been teaching yoga for six years at that time. I fell in love with yoga when I saw how it changed me and the other people that came to my classes. I watched as people began coming off their medications. I watched people achieve personal goals they had struggled with for years. I didn't understand the reasons and I didn't try to understand. I watched. I trusted.

After I was diagnosed with breast cancer, yoga was a place of acceptance for me. Yoga accepted me, where I was each time I got on the mat. I learned that each practice would be different. I might be able to do a headstand one day but the next day it wasn't a good choice for me. I learned that some days I needed a vigorous practice and some days I needed peace. It was hard for me to believe that I needed to listen to my body and not my mind during cancer.

Yoga didn't demand that I be perky or keep a smile plastered on my face. Yoga didn't care what size my jeans were, how I wore my hair or the kind of car I drove.

Yoga was a place where I was just another yogi. These yogis were my family. I didn't have to be anything I was not. No one cared that I was going through cancer treatments. No one cared that I was bald. No one cared that I wore a wig or took it off and shook it out when I got too hot. Yoga was an escape for a short time from the anxiety I was going through. Yoga met me where I was each day, but I never left the mat the same.

The students that came to my classes at the gym loved me, prayed for me and worried about me. On the mat we were all one. We were all the same. We were all healthy. We were all stressed. We were all sick. We were all broken. We were all healed.

When I entered the classroom to teach yoga during my cancer treatments, I entered with stress, fear, and anxiety. Each time I exhaled, I exhaled all my concerns – at least for that one hour.

Yoga was not a magic pill. It was not a cure-all for what ails you but for me it was an escape from things I didn't want to face all the time. It was a place to be quiet, to be still, to be introspective.

It was hard for me to be alone with my thoughts. It was hard to stomach the fact that I had cancer and could die.

I could have died and not seen my children grow up.
I could have died and not been there to make sure they were loved.
I could have died and not accomplished the things I wanted to accomplish.
I could have died and not known what it was like to truly be loved.

I didn't die. I am alive, and I am healthier than I have ever been. I am healthier physically and I am healthier emotionally.

Yoga did not save me, but yoga helped me to save myself.

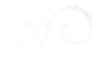

Buttermilk

All daddies should make their daughters feel like a princess. I felt like a princess with two feet solidly on the ground. I felt loved.

I was born at Fort Rucker, Alabama when my father was in flight school, learning to fly L-19 airplanes, the first of many airplanes and helicopters he would learn to fly. He was an Army Master Aviator. We moved to Centerville, Tennessee when I was a baby. My mom liked to say I was born in L.A. – Lower Alabama. She loved being an Army wife. She loved being married to my dad. My mother was only 20 years old when I was born, and my dad was 23.

We moved around often when I was a child. We moved to Mineral Wells, Texas when I was 2 years old and my father learned to fly helicopters. We moved to Los Angeles, California when I was 5 years old and my father went to graduate school at UCLA. When I was 8 years old we lived in Alexandria, Virginia for 6 months while Dad was at the Pentagon and we moved to Arlington, Virginia when I was 12 years old for a year when he went back to the Pentagon.

My mom loved the D.C. area. We would get home from school and she would take us on an adventure. We explored the Smithsonian weekly. We visited the Capital, Mount Vernon and the monuments. We took advantage of everything the area offered. Washington, D.C. was our playground. We did not take it for granted. The last time we moved for the military, I was 13 years old.

Fort Leavenworth was located outside of Kansas City and in order for my dad had to attend Command and General Staff College we moved again. We lived outside of Fort Leavenworth in Platte City, Missouri. I cried all the way to Missouri. I didn't want to leave my friends. I didn't know if anyone in Missouri would like me. Mom told me something on that drive that stuck with me. She said, "No one knows you here. You can be whoever you want to be. No one knows you are shy". That comment didn't change me into a confident extrovert, but it did give me the belief that everything would be ok.

The military moved us around several times, but we always came back to Centerville until we moved to Nashville when I was in 8th grade. My father had grown up in Centerville and owned several businesses with his parents. That was our home base. One of the constants in my childhood was my pony; she was always there when we came home. We had wonderful people that took care of her when we were gone. Buttermilk was a birthday gift for my fourth birthday. I don't know that I would have remembered all the details of Buttermilk's arrival if they had not brought her home in the back of our blue station wagon. It never dawned on me that was an odd way to bring a pony home. I was born on January 8th, so I often got Merry Christmas/Happy Birthday gifts from other relatives. My parents always went out of their way to make a big deal over my birthday instead of lumping it in with Christmas. My pony was the best present I ever received for a birthday. Buttermilk was a huge part of my childhood. She was a part of my life from age 4 until we moved to Nashville when I was 13. I always thought I would have a horse.

When I went through my cancer treatments I often thought of my childhood. Children are free; free of fear, free of stress and free of the knowledge of your own mortality. There is a kind of peace you can find when looking into the eyes of a horse. The memory of Buttermilk's eyes eased much of my fear while I was waiting on the results of my mammogram.

The Mammogram

October 2006

The exam is over, and I am waiting in an open-front gown for the radiologist to read the mammogram. I wonder why they make me wear that gown. Blue, butt ugly print…1000 people have probably worn it. My arms don't fit in it right. There are snaps on the shoulders. It is misshapen, and it seems like there is always a boob trying to escape. No protection. All of my nerves exposed. No room for modesty.

I sit in the exam room reading Redbook. The magazine is three years old but there is an article on the front about how to lose 10lbs by walking 30 minutes a day. I have to read it; it could possibly contain the magic formula for weight loss. I wait. I wait. And I wait. It always feels like an eternity when you are waiting in a dimly lit exam room, in a bad gown, reading an old magazine about weight loss.

The radiologist doesn't come tell me himself. He sends the radiology technician in to tell me. She walks in slowly. She doesn't have a purposeful gait anymore. She doesn't hurry in to send me on my way. She looks sad. She carries pity in her eyes. I hate the look of pity. I watch as she processes what she is going to say and how she is going to say it. I wonder if they have a booklet for healthcare professionals called, "How to Give Bad News 101 Different Ways". I don't make it easy for her. I am still holding onto hope. Hope that maybe she looks worried because she is running late or needs a diet coke. Surely, she is worried about something else, something that has nothing to do with me. I sit.

I wait. Then she says it. We saw a mass; it might be nothing, but we need to schedule you for a biopsy.

Fear.

Stress.

Anxiety.

My kid's faces.

Nothing.

I am sitting in my car in the parking lot of the hospital. I don't remember walking through the lobby. I have the card with the date and time on it in my hand. I don't remember scheduling the biopsy. I remember sitting in the car and going nowhere. I remember my head hurting. I remember not being able to breathe in enough air. I remember needing my Mom.

Yoga for Fear

Yoga will relieve your fear. Really? It will not but it will help you better cope with fear.

Try alternate nostril breathing before you begin this flow.

Beginning in an easy seated position, focus on your breath. As you breathe in, say to yourself, *I am* … as you exhale, say to yourself, *calm*. Continue breathing like this for as long as you would like. Slowly move onto your hands and knees for Cat/Cow pose. Continue moving through the poses while focusing on your inhalations and exhalations. Breathing in, *I am* and exhaling, *calm*.

Affirmation– I am Calm

Poses:
Cat/Cow -
Downward Facing Dog
Plank – modified and/or full
Side plank
Forward Fold with Ragdoll arms (modification, knees bent)

Cat/Cow helps to get your body moving. I love the feeling of waking up the torso. In Cow pose I breathe in strength and in cat I exhale fear. Downward Facing Dog and Plank remind me that I am strong. Side Plank keeps me balanced and Forward Fold allows me to release the fears. These poses can be done individually, or you can repeat them in a flow. In a flow, you can rest in Downward Facing Dog between each pose.

Yoga For Fear

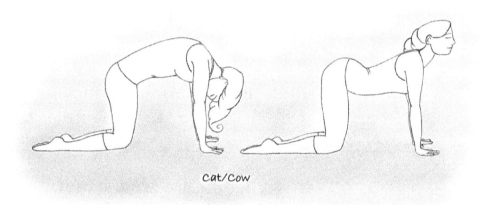

Cat/Cow

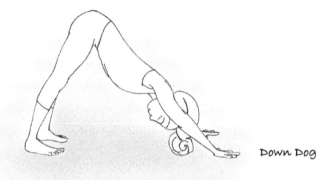

Down Dog

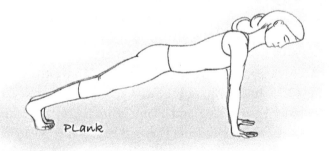

Plank

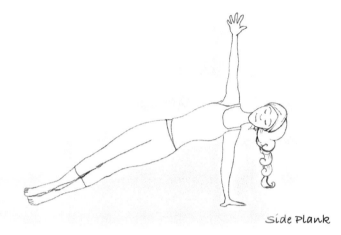

Side Plank

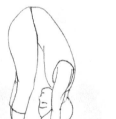

Forward Fold

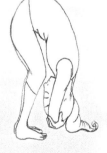

Ragdoll

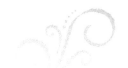

Breathing and the Ujjayi breath

I talk about breathing in all my yoga classes. It is a foundational piece in our yoga practice. It should also be a foundational piece in dealing with cancer.

We seldom think about our breath, though many of us do not breathe efficiently. I notice this in fitness classes when people struggle to breath and find themselves breathing shallowly. Creating an awareness of how we are breathing promotes better breathing. In yoga, we use our breath to help us in our yoga practice.

One of the first yoga trainings I did was with Beth Shaw's YogaFit. The trainer stated that it is common for us to only use the top 1/3 of our lungs when we breathe. Shallow breathing can be caused by stress, tension or just habit. When we increase our oxygen intake it can give us more energy, increase concentration, improve mood and decrease stress.

I love it when a new student tells me they feel better when they walk through the doors of the studio and focus on their breath. Yoga breathing techniques can be done anywhere. Even just focusing your attention on your breath, without doing anything to change it, you move to a more relaxed place.

The first breath I teach in class is the ujjayi breath. The word ujjayi means victorious and it can be an energizing and a relaxing breath. This is an easy breath to master and has great benefits, lowers the heart rate, calms the mind, destresses and just makes you feel good. The key to this breath is relaxation.

- Sit in a comfortable position to learn this breathing technique.
- Breathe in and out deeply through your nose with your mouth closed.
- Inhale fully. Imagine sipping the breath in through a straw. If your inhale is too strong you would collapse the straw.
- As you exhale, you will have a soft humming sound in the back of your throat. You can hear yourself but someone across the room should not be able to hear you.
- You want to try to maintain the same breathing throughout your practice.

This is a creates a pleasing sound. This is the most common breathing technique used in yoga. The inhales and the exhales are calm and even. I tell my students that it may sound like the ocean in the back of the throat.

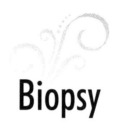

Biopsy

November 2006

"Here, put this gown on and leave it open in the front," the nurse tells me. I take off my clothes and neatly fold them and put them on the chair in the room. I put my bra between my pants and sweater, so no one will see it. I don't know why I always do that. I know they have seen bras before. The nurse said this will just feel like a hard pinch and I will be finished and, on my way, soon. I like the picture of the meadow on the wall. Why do medical offices always have the same pictures? The ones that are supposed to be pretty and calming. I stare at the picture, it was a cheaply framed reproduction of a Monet. The frame is plastic but designed to look expensive. Who buys this stuff? I look at the faint traces of a road in the high grass. I wish I was on that road or anywhere but here. "Are you ready," the nurse asks. It's cold … or is that fear shaking me from inside my body.

Oh my gosh! That didn't feel like a strong prick. It felt like someone took a knife held it over a fire then quickly jabbed the tip of it into my breast. I am lying on a table that has two holes in it for my breasts to fall through. I am in one of those dreadful gowns. I am lying face down with the doctor underneath the table. I am vulnerable. I am exposed. And I'm not supposed to move! I am scared. Please don't find anything. Please say it was nothing. Please be benign. Please. Please Lord.

Isn't there a better gown? One that is soft. One that doesn't scream "someone" else wore this. Is that "someone" ok? Is that "someone" still here? Does this gown hold some of those other patients' fears in its fibers? Why isn't there a different gown? Why aren't they done yet? Why do I have to try to be so strong? Why didn't I let someone come with me? Why didn't anyone insist on coming with me? Why didn't my husband realize I needed him today?

I am alone…in this gown.

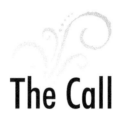

The Call

The phone was going to ring. I could feel it. I could feel the energy in the back room of our store. My heart was like those hearts you see in cartoons. It felt like it was beating out of my chest. It felt like there was a long pause in between beats. My heartbeat was in my throat. I couldn't breathe. I didn't know how much more of this I could take.

The nurse said they would call on Thursday. It was a Thursday. It was 5:00pm. Did they forget about me? I wanted them to call and relieve my stress. I didn't want them to call and confirm my fears. I wanted them to call and tell me it was nothing. I didn't want them to call and say the "C" word.

Call.

Don't call.

Call.

Don't call.

The phone rang. I didn't want to answer it. I felt the answer already. I didn't need to answer because I already knew.

Ring…

"Hello, this is Dr. Warren's nurse".

Why couldn't I breathe? Why couldn't I say hello back to this nice woman? Why did I just grunt out a strange sound, kind of like …lo? She was telling me she stayed late to get my test results. "I knew you would be worried and anxious to hear the results of your biopsy". She took a breath, "I am so sorry to have to tell you that the biopsy showed cancer".

I was numb. I thought this must be how it felt to be shot by a gun. Her words were the gun. My voice quivered. Why did I suddenly feel so fragile? I experienced a new kind of fear. The fear of the not knowing was gone. I felt as though I was watching this scene from another place, a safe place. A place where cancer doesn't exist.

I told her I wanted to see the surgeon as soon as possible and I wanted to have the surgery as soon as possible. She made me an appointment with the surgeon on the coming Tuesday.

She said there were no openings for the surgery, if that is what I decide to do, until after Thanksgiving. I couldn't wait that long. I couldn't have that in my body that long. She told me there may be an opening the next Friday if she moved a few things around.

I told her I would take it.

You need to talk to Dr. Warren first. "Ok, I'll talk to him on Tuesday and we can do the surgery Friday," I told her. She said ok. She said again that she was sorry. My voice trembled. I tried to force out a pleasant thank you and hang up. I sobbed. Could you call it sobbing if you had tears streaming down your face, but you weren't making any sound?

I didn't make sense as I tried to tell my husband what the nurse had said. I wanted him to hold me and comfort me and tell me I would be ok. I don't remember any comforting words he said that evening. I don't remember him holding me. I only remember how I felt. I always thought I was invincible. Cancer didn't happen to me. Cancer happened to other people. It was something I would read about but never encounter. Cancer was a death sentence. Cancer = Death.

I cried. I needed a tissue for my nose. What was I going to tell my kids? They would be so scared. They found out two months ago that their grandmother had pancreatic cancer. She was not doing well. I knew one thing: I didn't want to die.

Please hold me. Please tell me I am going to be ok. Please.

A Beautiful Soul - a poem

Most of my life I have heard – you are such a beautiful girl.
You have such a pretty face.
I look in the mirror – where is this girl they are talking about.
The woman I see looking back at me is insecure.
The woman staring right through me is scared.
She is lonely, terribly lonely.
She feels betrayed.
She feels she is to blame for causing pain.

When I look back into that mirror I see a woman
who has had to be silent to survive,
though it is not in her nature.
I see a woman who hates confrontation so much
that she has allowed herself to become a victim.
I see a woman who despises herself for allowing her soul to be victimized.

As I stand here in front of this mirror, I look closer.
I look deep into those hazel green eyes.
I am searching for the girl in the woman.

As I look into this woman's eyes, now I see hope.
I look closer – I see strength. In this strength, I see desire.
Desire for change. Desire for love. Desire for happiness.

I see the girl that used to live inside this woman. The girl that was told,
"If you would only lose a little weight you would be beautiful,
because you have such a pretty face".

I see the girl that was told by men she was pretty
only to be used and destroyed by them.
I see the girl who believed in love and hope and happiness.

I look closely at this beautiful girl and watch as she sheds
the burdens she has allowed to gather around her and pull her down.
I look closely, and finally I see beauty.

I see a beautiful soul.

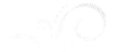

Yoga for Self-Acceptance

We all struggle with self-acceptance in some way. Being happy and satisfied with yourself helps you to find more joy in your life.

Affirmation: I am enough
Easy seat – lotus mudra – sit and breath for 8 slow inhalations.

The Lotus Mudra is a grounding mudra. It is a great way to focus on maintaining your foundation and when you have a strong foundation, you have a better chance at self-acceptance. Bring the base of the palms together at the heart center, touching the thumbs and pinky fingers together. Spread the rest of the fingers out like the lotus flower opening toward the sunlight.

Flow:
Child's pose flow – Child's pose, come up onto knees (shins on floor), reach arms to the sky, back to Child's pose, repeat 8 times
Downward Facing Dog
Warrior 1, right leg in front, arms out to sides, chest up to sky, inhale
Plank
Upward Facing Dog
Downward Facing Dog
Back to right leg in front
Open to Sun God
Warrior 1 to other side left leg in front, arms out to sides, chest up to sky, inhale
Plank
Upward Facing Dog

Downward Facing Dog
Child's pose
Repeat

The way you approach your practice effects the benefits you will reap. I chose these poses because of the way they make you feel mentally and physically.

Childs pose is a place to surrender the self-doubt, even if only for the time you are on your mat. Hopefully, you will remember how free you felt later when you are tempted to pick the self-doubt back up. The poses in this flow help you feel strong, balanced and in control. I love this flow when I want more love and compassion for myself.

Yoga For Self-Acceptance

Warm up to Surrender Self-Doubt

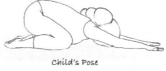

Child's Pose

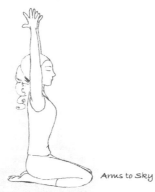

Arms to Sky

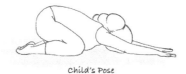

Child's Pose

Yoga Flow for Self-Acceptance

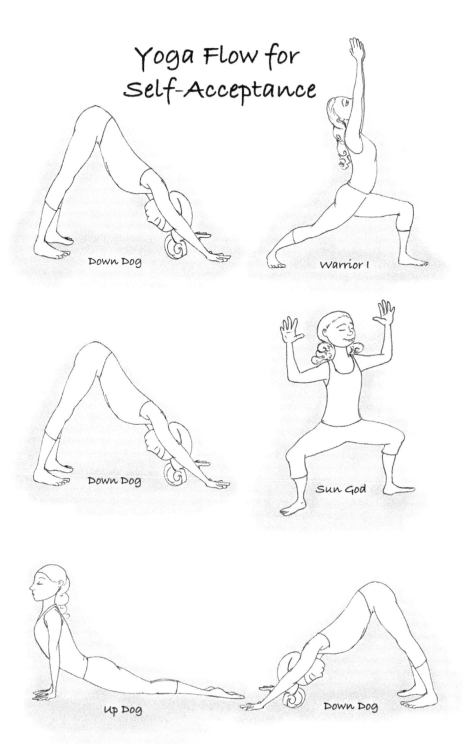

Down Dog

Warrior I

Down Dog

Sun God

Up Dog

Down Dog

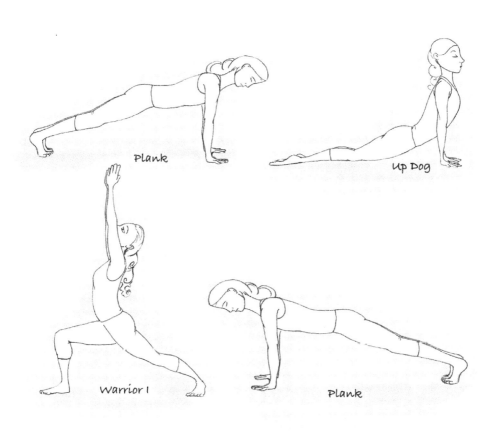

Plank

Up Dog

Warrior I

Plank

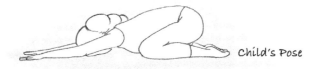

Child's Pose

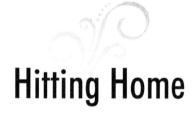

Hitting Home

How do you tell the people in your life you have cancer? You want them to know in order to comfort you and tell you that you'll be ok. You don't want to tell them because that means it's real.

The phone call…the nurse told me. My then husband, David, was there, so I told him. He tried. He did. He just never knew the right things to say. I have to believe that. I can't believe he didn't care or that I was going to be an inconvenience. He tried, right?

My children. I couldn't tell them, so David did. I still remember his exact words and theirs, "Mother is going to have surgery Friday. She has breast cancer."

Samantha and Mack assumed he was talking about his Mother (whom they called Mer). They didn't call me Mother, but he called his mom, Mother.

"Oh my gosh," said Samantha, "I can't believe Mer has pancreatic cancer and breast cancer."

"No," David said, "your mother has breast cancer."

I was sitting on the floor, trying to be strong and not cry. I couldn't look at their faces. I knew if I looked at them, I couldn't hold it together. Mack ran to his room and shut the door. Samantha went to her room and shut the door.

I couldn't move. I needed to be held. I was alone in the room with my husband. He didn't pull me up from the floor. He didn't tell me I was going to be fine. He didn't say anything.

I stopped crying. It couldn't just be about me now. I had to go check on Samantha and Mackenzie. The walk from the living room, through the kitchen and study wasn't that long but it felt like it took forever. I walked down the hall to Mack's room first. I opened his door. He was sitting on the edge of his bed with his feet up on the antique bedrails. He didn't look at me when I came in. He knew it would be me.

"Mackenzie? I said. Are you ok?"

He looked up at me with tears and fear in his eyes. I grabbed him into my arms. He cried. I cried.

"Ma, are you gonna be ok?"

"Of course, I am. You are my lucky charm."

"I'm scared Mama. I don't want you to die."

Mack was eleven years old. He was growing up, but that night he was just my little boy. He snuggled into my arms and let me hold him. After a few minutes, I told him I needed to go check on Samantha. He laid down on his bed and looked at the ceiling.

I slowly opened the door to Samantha's room. I expected her to be on her bed crying. I expected her to be devastated. She was both, but more than that, she was mad.

"Why didn't you tell me?" she cried.

"We just told you."

"No, Daddy told me," she said.

I knew what she meant. She wanted to know why she was finding out after the fact. She wanted to know why she wasn't asked to go with me. She wanted to know why she wasn't there to hold my hand, so I wouldn't be alone. She knew I had been alone.

"Samantha, I didn't know it was even going to be cancer. I didn't want to worry you if it was nothing," I told her.

"How did you find out? How long have you known?" she said softly through tears.

"I went in for my regular mammogram a couple of weeks ago. They saw a mass."

"A mass!" she shrieked.

"They saw a mass," I continued, "then they scheduled me for a biopsy. I got the results tonight."

"Did Daddy go with you for the mammogram and biopsy, so you didn't have to be alone?"

"No, he had to run the store, I was fine."

"I would have gone with you, Mommy. You didn't have to be alone," she said, sobbing.

She laid down on the bed in the fetal position and cried. She was sixteen years old but seemed so young that night.

"Are you going to be ok?"

"Yes."

"Are you scared?"

"Yes."

I held her tight.

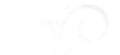

Van Halen

David came with me. He got me checked in for surgery at 6 a.m. and then he left. He took the kids to school. He went to open our store. He said he'd be back after the store was closed at 6pm. I told him I was scared of possibly needing a mastectomy; he said don't worry about that. If you need one, we'll get you some hooker boobs.

Who says that to their wife when she has breast cancer?

I was scared. Why was I there - alone? I would have rather been alone than with him on that day. But I was scared. Scared of the hospital. Scared of the surgery. Scared of the unknown. I wanted to know that I would be ok. I didn't want to know that I would not be ok. The surgeon plays Van Halen during the surgery. What does that mean?

When I met my surgeon and my lumpectomy was scheduled, I asked him what music he listened to when he was operating. He was caught off guard. He was a nice but reserved man. I could tell he didn't open up to others easily or at least not to his patients. When I asked about his music, he looked nervously around the room as his nurse laughed. I looked at him and said "don't tell me you play head banger music or hard rock when you are doing surgery!"

His nurse smiled and told me he listens to Van Halen. I looked at him and laughed. I said, "Well, you better bring me a shirt before we do this."

He did. The morning of my surgery, he walked in and threw me a Van Halen shirt.

The day of the surgery was long. There were delays. I wanted to get it over with, but I knew they would get to me as soon as they could. I worried about myself and I worried about the patient they were operating on that kept me delayed.

I remember the waiting and being alone. I remember feeling like I didn't matter.
I remember crying. I remember being cold.

I remember the pain of the all the things that must be done before the lumpectomy. I remember the IV insertion, the placement of the locator needle in my breast and the pain of the injection of the dye. No one warned me until I got there of the searing pain of that procedure. They had to inject dye to find the sentinel node. I remember having to lie still as they did it. I remember tears streaming down my face as I fought to hold still. I remember feeling scared and so very alone. I remember needing to pee. I always have to pee when it isn't convenient. Lying in the hospital bed, in that gown, with an IV. All I can think about is I have to pee.

My surgery was supposed to be at 7:30 a.m. It is 11a.m. I was still alone. They were not expecting the delay, so they did not have a place to put me. I was in a makeshift hospital room with a big needle sticking out of my breast.

That was where Carol and Michele found me. I had never been so glad to see anyone in my life. My two dear friends: Carol the nurse and Michele the yogi. Carol is the practical one that tells me to chill out, I'll be fine. I could see in her eyes that she was scared for me. Michele was the mothering, crazy-fun one that cried with me. She was scared for me too. They were here. I was not alone. They made me laugh. "Why do you have a wire sticking out of your boob?" "Why do you keep going to pee? You just went." They hugged me. I was not alone.

The operating room personnel came for me. They rolled me towards surgery. The nurse smiled at me and told me how lucky I was to have Dr. Warren for my surgeon. He is the best. The room was so cold. Why was it so bright? I didn't hear Van Halen. I guess he waited until I was out before he turned on the music. There were so many people in there. The anesthesiologist was telling me to count backwards from ten.

I needed to go to pee.

Nuclear Medicine - a poem

I wear the gown when I go to nuclear medicine.
The gown is not there for me.
No one is there for me.
Who is no one
Who are you
You are not my mother
My mother loves me
Love is not real
Aggression is real
Cancer is aggressive
Cancer can be stopped with money
I hate money
Hate not knowing who I am now
Who am I
I write
I rhyme
Rhyming is how the world works
I wear a Nuke gown.
I wear the gown when I go to nuclear medicine.

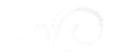

Blue Dye

Nuclear medicine was a stop I had to make on the way to surgery. I had not been told about this until I was wheeled in to this department. It was explained to me that they would be injecting nuclear dye in several spots around the tumor. This would help them find the sentinel node, so they would have to take out less lymph nodes. The entire day was traumatic, but this was painful. The breast area is sensitive anyway and especially the nipples, so it was not surprising this would be a bit painful. The nuclear technologist asked me if I had been told it would be painful and I told her I was told it was a little uncomfortable.

It was more than uncomfortable. It was not expected. I am still not sure why I wasn't warned and why I had never heard how painful this was. It is hard to describe how the injection of the nuclear dye felt. It burned. It felt the way I imagined it would feel to have acid poured on your breast.

The technician was a young girl with a soft voice and comforting eyes. She told me I had to be still. She said there would be pain. I was not prepared.

Yoga for after Breast Cancer Surgery

After you have surgery for breast cancer you may have a decrease in the range of motion in your arm and shoulder. This will vary depending on if you have a biopsy, lymph node biopsy, lumpectomy, mastectomy and/or breast reconstruction. You will not want to do any of these exercises without first getting permission from your doctor. Remember, you need to always listen to your body when you exercise. Start slowly. Add poses as they feel comfortable.

Affirmation: I am whole
Poses:

Mountain to Forward fold. Add, standing backbends as you flow. Repeat 8+ times.
Add Eagle pose on each side when you get ready to change sides
Add Crescent Lunge after the Eagle on each side.

Take your time. Full inhales and exhales in each pose before you add the next.
As you feel more comfortable, open arms to sides and lift chest in crescent.

Flow through these poses until you feel ready to move to Downward Facing Dog. Notice how you feel in Downward Facing Dog.

Move to the floor. Focused breath for 2 minutes.

Cow Face Pose
Savasana
Mountain pose is a strong grounding pose. You need that after surgery. Stay in this pose for several breaths. Forward Fold is a nice releasing pose for me. I love to dive towards the floor and release the worries and tension. Eagle pose helps to feel balanced though you may not be able to add the arms soon after surgery. The concentration required for Eagle is great to help take you mind off the surgery. The arms are moving to the midline of the body, so this pose should be accessible.

Downward Facing Dog helps to remind you that you are strong but remember to listen to your body. Cow Face pose will help you start working on your range of motion after surgery, make sure you are take your time moving deeper into this pose.

Yoga after Breast Cancer Surgery

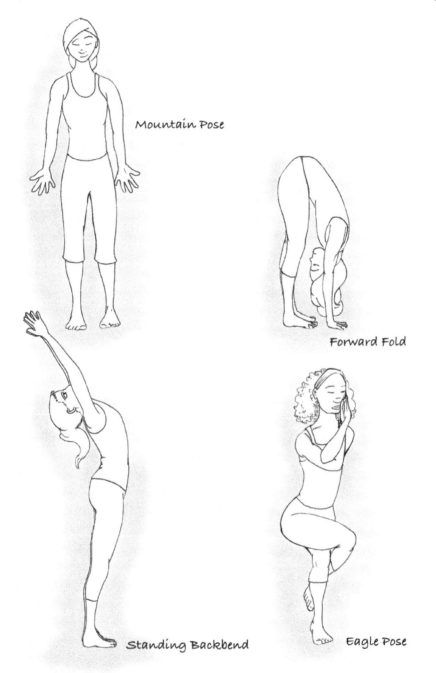

Mountain Pose

Forward Fold

Standing Backbend

Eagle Pose

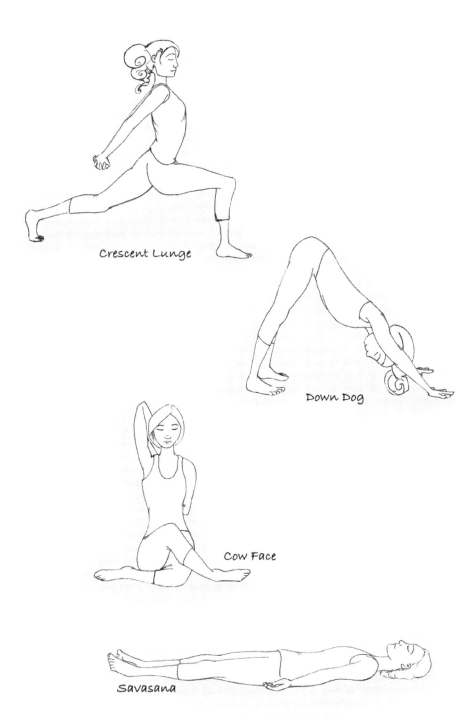

Crescent Lunge

Down Dog

Cow Face

Savasana

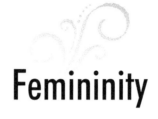

Femininity

Most women are recognized as women by the way they look. Their breasts. Their hair. Their figure. This is the foundation of femininity.

Much of my life I have been embarrassed about my breasts. I was self-conscious about how large they were. I tried to find minimizing bras and shirts that did not draw attention to my breasts. I fought against that part of me for much of my pre-cancer life. My hair was another part of me I struggled with. I never had the long straight hair that I thought was pretty. I had wild, uncontrollably thick, curly hair. I never saw anyone on television or in magazines with hair like mine.

Having breast cancer was very hard. To have it effect the other part of me I had also fought with was doubly hard. In truth, my breasts and hair were the two parts of my body that defined my appearance.

I was 11 when I realized I was getting breasts. I remember how nervous I was when I told my mother I needed a bra. We didn't talk about those kinds of things. I was in sixth grade and probably should have started wearing a bra in the fourth grade. I remember the boys giggling and pointing because I didn't have that telltale outline of a bra on my back. The outline that told the world I was getting older.

"Mommy, I think I should maybe… or we should…could…," I stammered.

"What, Cathleen?" she said as we drove into town. We were not often alone. I was the oldest of four children and it was rare that I had my mother to myself.

"I wonder if we could go get me a…. bra," I whispered.

"Ok," she said. I was so relieved. I didn't have to tell her I wanted that outline on my clothes so the pointing would stop. If I had known it would have been this easy, I would have asked a long time ago.

We went to the only store in town that carried bras. Mom walked me in and told the sales lady what we needed. "We will need to measure her," she said. She got out her tape measure and wrapped it around my chest in three places. She made a big deal out of the whole procedure. I felt so grown up but also embarrassed.

"She should have been in here before this," she announced. The sales lady walked away and came back with two boxes. Each box contained a different size training bra. I wondered what my breasts were going to be trained to do. Were they being trained to grow? Were they being trained to not grow? Were they being trained to leap over tall buildings in a single bound?

It felt weird wearing a bra. I didn't feel free anymore. I felt managed. I was under control. I took off the bra and began putting it neatly back into its box as the sales lady whipped back the curtain and demanded to see it on me. I was mortified standing there topless as she helped me put the bra back on. She adjusted the straps, tightened the band around my chest and announced we had a perfect fit. I started to take the bra off and she said, "Just give me the box and you can wear the bra home." I was thrilled. I came out of the dressing room beaming. I had my first bra.

The attention to my breasts was not something I desired. I wanted people to see me, not my breasts. When I was in seventh grade we moved to Platte City, MO. My dad was stationed at Fort Leavenworth, KS for Command and General Staff College. We were only going to be there for six months. I was terrified. I was going to begin junior high school, which was a big deal all by itself, but to move to Missouri added even more stress. I worried and fretted all the way from Tennessee to Missouri.

"What if no one likes me?" I asked. "What if I don't have any friends?"

"You will have friends, you always have friends," said my mother. "Cathleen, no one in this new school knows anything about you. They don't know you are shy. They don't know you are scared. You can be anyone you want to be. Think about the girls in Centerville that you wanted to be like. Here, you can be anyone you want to be."

I had to mull that one over, but it gave me a new confidence I had never had before. I was still shy. I was still scared but I had something to consider. Could it really be that easy?

The first week of school there was an announcement for cheerleading tryouts. I signed up. I tried out in front of the whole school. I made it. To this day, I can't believe I tried out and was chosen to be a cheerleader. Platte City was a small town. I was the new kid; maybe that was why I was chosen. In one of the first football games of the season we played the neighboring county. One of the cheerleaders ran up to me and said the guys on the other team were asking who the new cheerleader was. I was flattered when she said, "they said you were pretty". I was deflated when she added, "and has big boobs." What was it about these two blobs on my chest that drew so much attention? This is probably the point where I could have decided to use these things as a super power, but I didn't. I became more self-conscious.

My breasts grew a little more after seventh grade and seemed to slow down by high school, "thank you Lord". We moved back to Tennessee after six months in Missouri. We moved to Nashville for my eighth-grade year, this was the final move of my Dad's career. I went to school in Nashville then changed schools for my last two years of high school. I made cheerleading again in eleventh and twelfth grade in my new school. I loved my school in Lebanon, Tennessee. I did not even mind the forty-five-minute drive each way. My favorite part of going to a private co-ed school was that we wore uniforms to school. Girls had two options: pants with a gray shirt or a plaid skirt with a white shirt. When the weather was cool the girls wore V-neck navy sweaters with our skirts. I had read that a V-neck was more flattering on girls with larger breasts. It felt safe. The button-up shirts had to be roomy enough, so they would not have a gap in the front. I didn't have breasts that were abnormally large - I wore a 34C bra. They weren't dangerous to the passerby. They just drew attention and I didn't like that kind of attention. No one treated me differently – probably because I wasn't the circus sideshow that I had felt I was. There was only one time that I felt self-conscious at my high school. We had a school radio station that played music during lunch and after school. One afternoon I was staying late for cheerleading practice and over the loud speakers came a request for me. Someone had requested the song, "Brick House" by The Commodores. It probably had nothing to do with my breasts. I wore sweaters for a week to try to disappear.

After high school there didn't seem to be the same fascination with my breasts. I began not focusing on them because no one else seemed to be. When I walked into the classroom in college, there was no spotlight or warning lights announcing my breasts and I were entering the room. I just walked in and sat down.

Twenty-six years later...

"You have breast cancer" Cancer in my breasts. The part of my body that I most tried to hide.

I fought my body most of my life. I dieted and exercised to lose weight. I tried to minimize my breasts with special bras. Going through cancer diagnosis and treatments changed the way I look at my body and my hair. I don't think I'll ever be completely happy with my body size, but I am happy that I'm alive. I don't think I will ever want to show off my breasts, but they are now healthy. I don't complain about a bad hair day anymore – I have hair.

Beating myself up because I didn't look a certain way, was exhausting. It took time away from happiness and a full life. I found more joy in my life when I quit focusing on my flaws and appreciated my life.

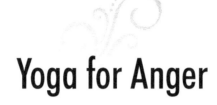

Yoga for Anger

Anger and fear took turns being in charge during this time. I was scared then I was angry. I was scared that I would not be okay. I was angry that I had done everything right and I still got cancer. I ate right, and I exercised. Wasn't that supposed to keep me healthy? My rational side knew that cancer was random, but my irrational side was mad.

It is hard to hold anger and kindness in the same hand.
Affirmation: I am kind.

Sun Salutation A

- Mountain
- Forward Fold
- Monkey
- Plank
- Upward Facing Dog
- Downward Facing Dog
- Forward Fold
- Mountain

When you have exhausted your anger:
Seated Forward Fold, Easy Seat with a focus on your breath and finish with Legs Up the Wall Pose.

Sun Salutation A can be a complete practice alone. It can stretch, strengthen and relax the body. This practice can also reduce anger and stress. Sun Salutations are generally used to energize the body, but they can also be done in such a way that relaxes the body.

To do Sun Salute A: Begin in Mountain pose, breathe. Reach your arms up towards the sky, noticing how your body feels, Forward Fold. Release the back of the body and release the anger and fear. Flatten your back and hold your belly in as you move to Monkey pose. Step back into Plank or Modified Plank, lower your body down to Upward Facing Dog or Modified Cobra. Move to Downward Facing Dog, let your back body stretch. Remember, Downward Facing Dog is a resting pose, when you are ready, step back in to a Forward Fold then lift back up into Mountain Pose. Continue this flow until you are ready to move into Legs Up the Wall Pose.

Yoga for Anger

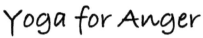

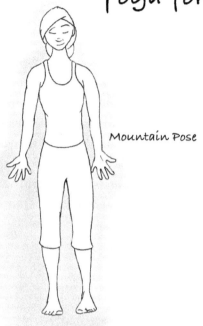

Mountain Pose

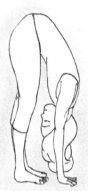

Forward Fold

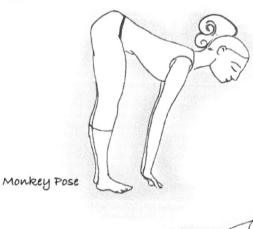

Monkey Pose

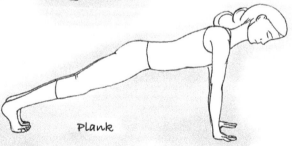

Plank

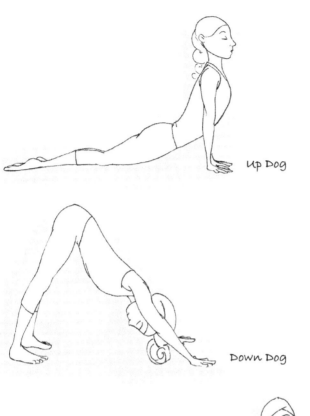

Up Dog

Down Dog

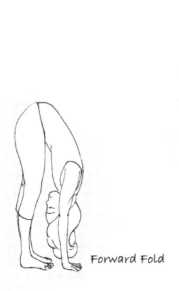

Forward Fold

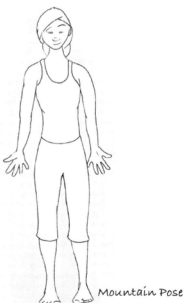

Mountain Pose

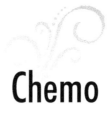

Chemo

January 4, 2007

Chemotherapy. Poison. You have to pump poison into my body? That is the best drug you have now to make sure all the cancer is gone? Poison - can heal me? Why is this the only treatment? Why isn't there a cure for cancer? I have to have more surgery to have a port, a permanent IV port, inserted into my body. Why does the surgery for the port hurt worse than the lumpectomy? When do I start chemo? Can I wait until after Christmas? I don't want to ruin Christmas for my kids.

January 4th. I walk slowly down the hall towards the large chemo room, a room with recliners and TV's attached to each recliner. I don't want to be in the big room. In the big room, there is group fear which is like group therapy, only more desperate. In the big room there are nurses administering chemo drugs, commiseration between patients, talk about dry mouth, where to find the best knit caps, how long the nausea, insomnia and fatigue last.

"Cathleen, you could help comfort them," the nurses tell me.

I don't want to. I want to be alone. Alone with my fear. Alone with my anxiety.

As I walk down the hall, I notice the meditation room on the right, an oasis on the way to the chemo room. I never go into the meditation room for fear it would mean all of my hope was gone but I am glad the room is there. I felt peace and calm just by passing it on the way to the poison.

46

The door to the chemo room is ahead of me. I have to be buzzed in. Why? Are they trying to keep people in or out? Out I guess. I don't have to be buzzed out. I slowly reach my hand out towards the door. I hear the buzz. I don't want to walk in. Do I have to? Why did today have to get here so fast? Will it hurt? Why isn't my husband holding my hand? Is he scared too?

It is 7:30 in the morning. I asked to be first. There are private rooms around the sides of the chemo room. Private rooms are on a first-come basis. I want to be alone. I don't know what to expect. I didn't ask. They would have told me if it was painful, right?

A nurse greets me. Her name is Maria. She walks me towards the recliners. "Can I please have a private room?" I ask. She holds my hand and says I can be wherever I feel the most comfortable. The room is nice, a recliner for me, a recliner for my caregiver, and a TV on the wall. Maria asks me to sit down. I have to have two different kinds of chemo.

She begins the Cytoxan first. I watch the clear poison move down the clear IV tube into my port. I can't take my eyes off of it. Maria tells me they are giving me steroids to help with the nausea and I will get a prescription for Zofran to help with nausea at home. I am not really listening to her. I am watching the poison. I glance out the window. There is a parking lot full of cars. Where are the people going? Are they going on with their lives while I am having chemo?

My husband is reading a book and watching Fox News. I wish he would talk to me.

The poison is now in my body. I don't feel different yet. I'm not nauseous yet.

Why is this happening to me? What if I die? Who will love my kids if I die? Will there be anyone to remind them how much I loved them? I sit there in silence. On the outside I'm still. On the inside I'm screaming. I'm scared and defeated. I am holding a book. I can't read. I can't pretend this is a normal day.

I don't remember how long it took for the chemo bag to empty. I thought both drugs would be in the same bag. Maria came back in to remove the first IV bag, she said she would return with the Adriamycin. I didn't understand that there was a difference. She came back with a huge syringe filled with bright red poison.

It looked like death. Bright red, poison that could eat away my skin if it got on me. I asked her why she wasn't going to hook it up like the Cytoxan and she said she had to manually administer the Adriamycin, slowly. I watched her for a few minutes. She sat beside me, with the poison. I looked away. I looked at my husband, across the room.

He looked up and said, "What's wrong?"

"Nothing," I choked out.

I laid my head back and looked out the window. Why am I crying? It doesn't hurt. Why are the tears rolling down my face? Normally, I would have been chastising myself for crying. But today, in the cancer center, in the chemo room, in the recliner, I let the tears flow. They flowed with fear. Fear for my own life. Fear for my children. The tears fell silently down my cheeks, I didn't want to be noticed. After a few minutes I noticed Maria. She had stopped administering the chemo. I looked up at her face. She was crying with me. She held my hand and told me to let her know when I wanted her to begin again. I waited. There were no more tears – for now. Maria smiled at me and finished her work.

The cancer center was such a scary place but people like Maria eased the fear. As she finished, Samantha came running into the room. She took off from school to come check on me. She saw the fear on my face and hugged me. She squeezed herself into the recliner with me.

Another thing they don't tell you – when you go to the bathroom after having Adriamycin – you pee red.

Hugging the Porcelain Throne

I sat beside the toilet on a pallet I made in the floor of the bathroom. I had hugged the toilet throwing up a couple of times in college. Hugging the toilet and throwing up poison was so much worse. I hate throwing up anytime but knowing I was throwing up after a dose of poison was scary.

During chemo, steroids were in the IV bags, but for home, they gave me a prescription for Zofran. The nurse told me I'd feel fine for the next 24 hours but to get the prescription filled because I would need it after that. I filled it. There were a myriad of thoughts running through my mind. When would I get sick? Would I get sick? Does the chemo still work if I throw it all up? Yes, I knew this one made no sense but nonetheless, it was dancing around in my fear.

I felt queasy less than 24 hours after my first chemotherapy. It is hard to explain that feeling. It wasn't the feeling I expected. I just felt wrong. I took the Zofran as directed. I still got sick. I was thankful for the Zofran. If I had not had that, I was sure it would have been worse. David, Samantha and Mack were all home the first time I got sick. David brought me a glass of water and asked if I needed anything else.

"No, but thank you," I said.

Samantha and Mack followed me into my bathroom when they saw me running. "You guys leave your Mom alone. Go to your rooms," David told them.

Mack went to his room but came back every 15 minutes or so to check on me.

Samantha said, "I'm going to get a cool washcloth for Mommy." David said ok. Samantha came back into the bathroom with a cool cloth, her book and a pillow.

"I'm staying here with you. What else do you need," she asked?

"Nothing. I'm fine," I said through tears.

I don't know why I couldn't quit crying. Maybe it was the emotion of the experience, the fear I felt for myself and my children, or the drugs, or maybe all of it. I stayed by the toilet for hours. Samantha stayed with me. I didn't want to be alone and I didn't want to have to lean on her so much. It didn't matter what I wanted then. I couldn't do much but throw up. I didn't make her leave; she wouldn't have gone anyway. She rubbed my back. She gave me cool cloths. She told me she loved me.

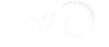

Yoga for Nausea

When you feel nauseous, the last thing you want to do is move around a great deal. The poses in this flow are meant to relax and relieve your body.

Affirmation: I am grounded

Poses:

Easy Seat

Bound Angle

Legs Up the Wall

Easy Seat is a hip opener and helps to reduce stress and anxiety.

Bound Angle stretches the inner thighs, groins and knees. This is another hip opener, so you can the same stress reduction benefits that you get in easy seat.

When I first started learning to teach yoga. I head from numerous instructors say that the hips were the emotional depot of the body, so releasing your hips helped to relieve a myriad of challenges to include, stress, anxiety and depression. I noticed, in my classes, that it had to a positive effect on my students. If we think about it when we feel stress, a normal reaction might be to curl ourselves into the fetal position. This movement is initiated in the hips and they tighten. So, stretching and releasing can help you to let go of that tension and stress.

Legs Up the Wall pose looks like a passive pose but it actually an active pose. Most everyone can do this pose, it doesn't require loads of flexibility and strength. This is one of my favorite poses. These poses help to relax you, improve your circulation, can help reduce swelling and it stretches your hamstrings and back.

Yoga for Nausea

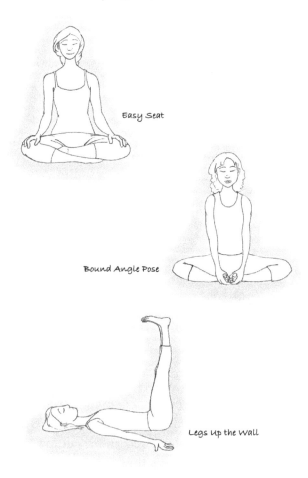

Easy Seat

Bound Angle Pose

Legs Up the Wall

What is meditation?

Meditation was the hardest part of yoga for me for years. I always thought I was doing it wrong. I had this vision in my mind of what meditation was and how it was done. I was not able to achieve this unrealistic ideal. I pictured yogis sitting with a clear mind. When I sat in mediation I had a myriad of things floating in an out of my mind. Breathing. Breathing. Breathing. I wonder what I should fix for dinner. Stop. Focus. Breathing. Breathing. What was that sound? Breathe. Breathe. You get the idea. I didn't realize then that I was still meditating. I was doing a great re-focusing meditation.

Meditation is a deliberate way of slowing down. There are few opportunities to just sit quietly is the fast pace of modern life. Meditation is easy, and you do not need any special equipment. All you need is a quiet place to sit and the desire to try.

To get started:

- Find a comfortable place to sit.
- If you can make this a regular part of your day it is easier to make it a habit. So, try to choose the same time.
- Loose or comfortable clothes.
- Turn off your phone. I often use my phone as a timer, so I put it on airplane mode.
- Decide ahead of time how long you are going to meditate and follow through.
- Try not to meditate on a full stomach.
- Sit with good posture.

- I like to rest my tongue lightly on the roof of my mouth as I breathe through my nose. I take a few deep breaths before I start to consciously relax my body.
- Remember to get rid of expectations about what you are supposed to be doing and just be, as you are.
- Close your eyes and focus on your breath.

There are some great mediation apps you can try to help. I like insight timer.

What Do You Say?

Cancer is evil. It is ugly and vile. It is more feared than a dark alley, snakes, or spiders. They aren't even in the same league.

People don't know what to say to someone with cancer. I didn't know what to say before I had cancer and I'm often not sure what to say now. I had a sweet lady come up to me after my diagnosis and ask me how long I had to live.

Everyone responds differently after they get a cancer diagnosis. There is fear but the way people live after a cancer diagnosis is different. I responded to my cancer diagnosis by staying even busier than I had been before. I was afraid to slow down. I was afraid to ask for help. I was afraid to let it sink in that … I had cancer. I still struggle to say that.

Looking back now I know I stayed busy because if I slowed down or asked for help, I would have fallen apart. I would have had to acknowledge that I had cancer and I preferred to deny the disease. In my mind, acknowledging it gave cancer more power over me. I was not sick. I did not want to be pitied or treated as if I was dying.

People often don't know how to react or what to do to help. I had a friend recently tell me she didn't ask if I needed her because I seemed so strong. She asked me what would have helped me when I was going through all the treatments. I thought about her question and before I realized what I was saying I said, "I would have loved someone to have come over, brought popcorn and a movie and made me sit down." I didn't slow down or sit down and I don't think I even exhaled at all during the seven months I was going through surgery, chemotherapy and radiation. I am not sure I would have slowed down then but that is what I needed. I was surrounded by many wonderful friends during that time and it would have been harder to go through those months without those wonderful women. My daughter was my caregiver but I never wanted to put more on her so I kept much of my fear and needs to myself.

What did I need?
I needed someone to hold me.
I needed my breast cancer to be acknowledged but not pitied.
I needed to feel like I mattered.
I needed to feel like I was not an annoyance.
I needed to feel like I was not being ignored.
I needed a husband that acted me like he cared.
I needed to feel like I wasn't alone.

Alone.

I hesitate when someone asks me what to say to a person going through cancer. That's a hard question. Each person responds differently and needs something different. It is important to let them know you care, and to let them know you recognize they are going through something scary. It is important to tell them they matter and are not being dismissed as if already dead.

Then, they don't feel quite so alone.

Yoga for Sleep

Many cancer patients experience problems sleeping during and after treatments. I was sleepy for about three days after chemotherapy and exhausted during radiation treatments. I was never a person that took naps, but I would find myself falling asleep if I ever slowed down during the day. The treatments took so much of my strength and disrupted my sleep. I was tired, but I struggled to fall asleep.

Poses:

Easy Seated Forward Fold

Child's pose

Legs Up the Wall

Lying Spinal Twist

Relaxation

Easy Seated Forward Fold is an easy pose to get into, opens the hips and relaxes the body. Forward fold can relieve headaches, lower stress and help with insomnia. Child's pose just feels good. There are several ways to do child's pose. You can find the best variation for you. Legs Up the Wall pose is one of my favorite yoga poses. It helps to improve circulation, relieve headaches and is considered a gentle inversion. This pose helps to relax the body, and this makes it easier to relax the mind. When our body and mind are relaxed we have a better chance of sleeping well. Lying Spinal Twist relieves tension in the back and helps digestion.

You may also want to try alternate nostril breathing for sleep.

Yoga for Sleep

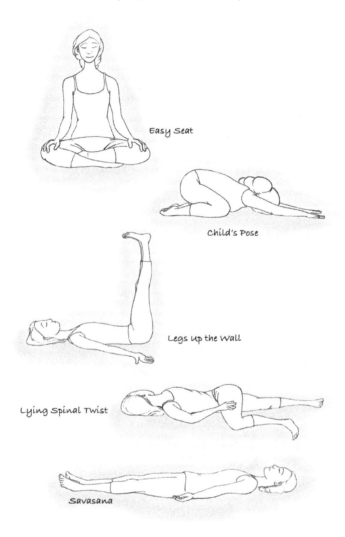

Easy Seat

Child's Pose

Legs Up the Wall

Lying Spinal Twist

Savasana

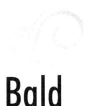

Bald

Dr. Cobos said some people on chemo don't lose their hair. He also said that chemo patients on Adriamycin and Cytoxan always lose their hair – all their hair. I didn't want my hair to fall out. Who would I be without my hair? My hair had defined me my whole life.

The day after my first chemotherapy, I had my long hair cut to shoulder length, a week later cut to chin length, then a day later cut into a pixie cut. I wanted some control over how I was going to lose my hair.

I quit thinking about bad hair days when they told me my hair would fall out on day ten. Ten days after I had chemo for the first time. On day ten, I sat on the side of the bathtub looking at myself in the mirror. I looked the same. Maybe tired and worried but outwardly, I looked the same. On the inside, that is where I had changed. I had aged. I had lost the belief that everything would always be ok.

I sat and contemplated my next move. If I took a shower and washed my hair I knew I would lose a lot of it. If I only took a bath and tried not to touch my hair very much – maybe I would have hair for another day. Every time I touched my hair, hair fell out. When I woke this morning there was hair on my pillow. There was hair on my shoulders throughout the day. It had begun falling out 3 days ago.

I sat on the side of the bathtub trying to decide if I wanted to just do it or delay it. It was going to happen. I was going to lose my hair. I was going to be bald.

I could not stop my hair from falling out. I could not make the follicles stay anchored in place. I could control when, where, and how I would lose my hair. I could control who would be with me when I lost my hair. Now was the only time I was strong enough to do it. I stood up; turned on the shower. I made the water hot, scorching hot. I needed to feel my body and know I was alive. I stood in the shower looking at the showerhead, knowing I was alive.

My chest rose and fell with my breath. I got my head wet. I could feel the water running down my back. I could feel my hair falling to the drain. I looked down at the floor of the shower. I stopped breathing. Within 30 seconds the floor was covered with hair.

My hair. What people had always admired about me. My hair. My shield from criticism because my hair was a part of me that usually didn't bring criticism. My hair, on the floor, not on my head. I slowly reached up to see if it was all gone. I still had hair! Maybe only some of it fell out. Maybe I would look the same, the same only with thinner hair. I grabbed the shampoo quickly. Washed the hair that remained. I couldn't wait to get out of the shower to see if I looked the same. Maybe I would be the exception. Maybe I wouldn't lose all of my hair. I grabbed a towel for my head. I slowly walked to the mirror. I took the towel off my head.

I screamed.

I quickly covered my head again. My daughter came running into my bathroom. She looked at me and hugged me tight. She held me as I cried. She rubbed my back and said, "It's ok Mommy". She was 16 years old. We switched roles at that point. She was the mother, I was the child. She held me until I quit shaking. She told me I was strong. She told me I was beautiful. She told me I was her hero. She told me she would always be there.

Slowly I stood up. Samantha was taller than I. She said, "Mommy, let me see". We took the towel off my head. She looked at me, started crying too and said, "It's just hair Mommy. You are still my beautiful Mommy".

I looked in the mirror at my eyes. Was I still there? There was only hair in a few places now on my head. Most of it was on the shower floor. I went to scoop it up. She said, "stop Mommy, I'll do it later".

I looked back at my eyes. I was still there. I thought I would see hopelessness. What I saw shocked me – I saw strength and the desire to remain strong. I had to be strong. I couldn't fall apart. I sat down on a stool in the bathroom. Samantha shaved off the last scraggly strands.

We were both crying.

Yoga for Constipation

The treatments for cancer have many side effects. Some chemotherapy drugs and radiation can cause constipation. I dealt with this during chemo and radiation. These yoga poses helped me. Move into each pose and stay there as long as it feels good to you. If you need a time, stay with each pose for 8 inhalations or more.

Affirmation: I am balanced

Poses:

Easy Seat Pose with deep breathing and/or meditation. You may want to add a twist to each side if that is comfortable.

Forward Fold, Ragdoll arms.

Downward Facing Dog

Lying spinal twist

Seated deep breathing and/or mediation helped to calm the stress and helped improve elimination. Forward fold calms the body and compresses the abdominal area. This can help with digestion. Downward facing dog is a full body stretch and helps to release tension. Lying spinal twist helps with bloating and gas. This pose is a great combination of a twist and a resting pose. Do each of these poses as a stand-alone. Stay with them as long as it feels good to you.

Constipation can happen anytime. I have found that I get constipated when I am stressed. Some chemotherapy drugs and some pain medication can have constipation as a side effect.

Yoga for Constipation

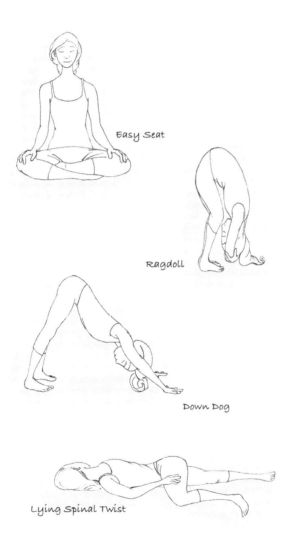

Easy Seat

Ragdoll

Down Dog

Lying Spinal Twist

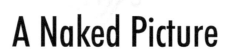

A Naked Picture

My head was always cold. I wore soft knitted caps. Not every cap would work, some were too tight, and some were scratchy. I saw a cancer patient when I saw my bald head.
I felt naked.

I felt fear. I rushed through my days pretending I was fine but when the wig came off and the reality of my cancer looked back at me from the mirror, I wondered if I would die. I wondered if I would be cured. Would I ever know what it was like to be loved for who I was under the hair? I wondered, what was my purpose for existing? Would I die and be forgotten, never having make a difference in the lives of others? I wondered how my kids would grow up without a mother. I wondered if they would forget how much I loved them. I wondered if they would forget me. I wondered so many things that it makes me cry even today writing about it.

I wanted to post a picture of me after I had lost my hair. I had not seen a picture of me with no hair since that time. I didn't know how I would feel to see me then. I went through all my external hard drives looking for pictures and I couldn't find any. I gave up; maybe there were no pictures chronicling my breast cancer journey. I had found a couple of me wearing a wig.

I mentioned to my son I had been looking for pictures of that time. He said, "I have one of you and Uncle Cliff." I was surprised. I am not sure how he ended up with one, but it was a relief to know there was a surviving picture. It was not hard to look at the picture of me even with no makeup, no sleep, nauseated and bald. It was hard to look at the mask I knew I was wearing. I could see in my eyes the fear and the exhaustion of trying to be strong.

During the time I was going through treatments, I was never bald in public. That would have been too much. I would have felt naked. People would occasionally ask me what I looked like bald and I would whip off my wig and show them. I acted as if my baldness didn't matter. I would laugh and announce, "Who knew I had a perfect shaped head under all that hair!" When I showed myself with no hair, I always waited for the reaction. I always wondered if I would shock people or would they see the real me without my hair. People always said I was beautiful without my hair when I did this, I just never believed them. My hair was my identity and it drew attention away from my insecurities.

I often talk about how I lost my hair and how it felt to have the part of me that had always defined who I was, gone in an instant.

What I've never really talked about how it felt to be bald. Being bald made me feel more vulnerable than I had ever felt. Being bald changed my life. I discovered I was more than my hair.

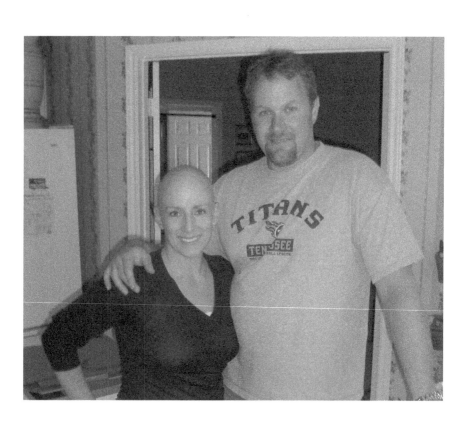

In The Fog — a poem

Standing in a thick fog.
Feeling uncertain where to turn.
Knowing there is something scary in the fog with me.
But not being able to move
out of the fog.

Chemo was my fog.
I was in the fog for three months.
They call it chemo brain.
I didn't feel bad
just not right.

Chemo every three weeks.
As soon as I would begin to see the fog lift
More chemo
more fog.

In the fog
I felt out of sorts.
Disoriented.

In the fog
I felt almost drunk.
not falling down drunk.
that disoriented drunk, right after tipsy.

In the fog

I just exist.
waiting for it to lift.
But know it will return.

In the fog
I am sheltered from painful memories.
I feel love and prayers
but I don't remember the words.

In the fog
there is a sick, kind of calm.

This is fear's home.

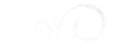

Yoga for Chemo Brain

Chemo brain, for me, was real and it was scary. I felt like I was living in a fog. I could not remember things. I had trouble focusing on what I was reading. My mind would wander, and I would have to re-read. Yoga may help with chemo brain, with your balance and with your memory.

For this flow use the Hakini mudra when you are in the poses. To do this mudra, bring your hands in front of your body, palms facing. Bring your fingertips of both hands together and allow them to lightly touch. This mudra helps with memory and concentration.

Affirmation: I am focused

Poses:

Mountain pose
Eagle, both sides
Chair pose
Crescent Lunge pose
Tree pose

Mountain pose makes you feel grounded. Eagle is a balancing and focusing pose. Chair pose helps you to feel strong. Crescent Lunge pose helps you to feel flexible and allows you to work on your balance. Tree pose is a balancing pose and a grounding pose. The intention of this pose it to feel strong, balanced and grounded.

Start in Mountain, breathe until you are ready to move. Slowly sit into Chair pose. Find your focus and balance before you move into Crescent Lunge pose. From Crescent Lunge, slowly move into Tree pose allowing your breath to move with your body. Breathe and balance, then move back to Mountain pose. Repeat other side

Flow through this short flow until you feel focused.

Move into meditation.

Yoga for Chemo Brain

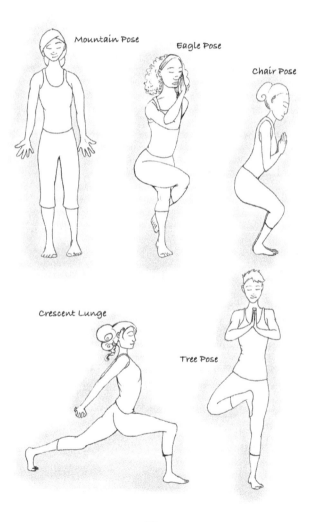

Mountain Pose

Eagle Pose

Chair Pose

Crescent Lunge

Tree Pose

Meditation for Chemo brain

Meditation can help relieve some of the challenges brought on by cancer treatments. All you need to meditate is a quiet place to sit, the ability to direct your attention, and a simple meditation technique.

Meditation is simple to do and doesn't require any special equipment. You can, however, prepare yourself and your space in a number of ways and make sure you have some basic amenities:

Comfortable place to sit and a position that is easy for you to maintain.

Phone turned off.

Willingness to try – you can't do it wrong.

Ujjayi breath - With this breath you make the breath audible but not loud. You make this breath just loud enough for only you to hear. This helps you to monitor the quality and quantity of the breath. It gives a focal point to your meditation and it just makes you feel good. Breath in deeply through your nose and as you exhale, create a soft humming sound in the back of your throat. You may feel that you sound a bit like Darth Vader, just make sure you are not that loud!

Sit in easy seat. Set a timer for 5-20 minutes. Find what will work for you.

Focus on your breath. Breath in and out deeply through your nose.

If you find you have thoughts or emotions drifting in, acknowledge them, and move back to the focus on your breath.

When your time is up. Bring your hands to your heart in an Anjali mudra. Breathe in and say to yourself, I am. Exhale and say to yourself, Focused.

Wigs

Rachel.
Phoebe.
Zoe.
Julia.

Weren't wigs for women that didn't want to "do" their hair every day? Or prostitutes? Or teenagers trying out new looks? Or Dolly Parton? Where do you even look for a wig store? Google. There was only one wig store in Lubbock, Texas. Wig Trend. It felt weird going to the wig store. The lights were that odd violet florescent. Where do I start? What color do I want? What style? I tried on wig after wig. The reason I was trying on wigs soon disappeared from my mind. It was fun trying on wigs. Being someone else, someone that didn't have cancer.

I found one wig that I liked more than the others. It was a little longer than shoulder length. It looked like Jennifer Aniston's hair. I bought it and called it Rachel. This was my serious wig. This was the wig I wore to church or special occasions. This would be the first wig I wore after chemo. This wig was tight. It felt confining. It wasn't long before I decided I needed a new wig. I needed a fun wig that I could wear when I taught aerobics - something different, something that wasn't tight.

Wigs itch on a baldhead. No one told me that either. I was finding out all sorts of things that people don't talk about. I never understood why more chemo patients wore hats than wigs. Wigs were uncomfortable, but wigs were safe. Wigs protected me from the stares of the normal people.

I went back to the wig store and found Phoebe. This wig was short and had attitude. It was dark auburn. The people in my fitness classes would cringe when I wore Phoebe. They knew class would be hard. Phoebe was my badass wig. This wig was lightweight, highly ventilated and sassy! I remember teaching aerobics and getting really sweaty. Off would come the wig. I shook it out, then put it right back on. I treated Phoebe like a hat.

I never felt like myself in the Rachel or Phoebe wig, so I made one final trip to the wig store.

I found my favorite wig, Zoe. This wig felt like me. The hair was shorter than I normally wore my hair. It was chin length and had long layers. It was wavy and red. It was me. This wig helped me to feel normal. This wig made me forget I was bald. I smiled from the inside.

As I was walking out of the wig store with my purchase (actually I wore it out,) I noticed a cute little blonde wig. It was a blonde bob. I don't know why I noticed a blonde wig. I had never wanted to be a blonde. Maybe I figured I had a brown wig, an auburn wig and a red wig, I needed a blonde wig to complete the collection of the versions of Cathleen. I tried it on. I bought it.

The first time I wore the blonde wig was to the gym to train a client. I felt awkward. It was blonde. As I walked in, one of the other trainers said, "Hey Cathleen, I love this one! You look like Julia Roberts."

I smiled, then stopped abruptly and asked, "You mean Julia Roberts in Pretty Woman when she was a prostitute?"

He looked flustered and said, "Well, yea. But you look like a classy prostitute".

Hmmmm … not the look I was going for. After that, I called the blonde wig Julia. I occasionally wore Julia when I felt unconventional.

Rachel. Phoebe. Zoe. Julia. These wigs protected me. Protected me from prying eyes. Protected me from stares. Protected me from pity. They made me feel normal, or as normal as I could feel then. When my hair started growing in several months later, I put my wigs in their boxes. This is where they stayed. I never gave them away. I didn't keep them because I thought I would need them again, or because they had become my friends or my protectors. I kept them because they are a reminder of a pivotal time in my life. They are a reminder of how different I am now. They are a confirmation that I am more than my hair.

Can I Get Cancer If I Hug You?

"Your head feels cool, Ma. I love you" said Mack as he rubbed my bald head.

When I was diagnosed with breast cancer, my kids were distraught. They gave me a lifetime worth of love in the months after my diagnosis. If I had doubt that I was loved in this life, they removed it.

"Can I get cancer when I hug you? Will you be ok? Are you going to be bald? I like your hair, Mama. Will it grow back if it falls out? Why will it fall out?" Mack asked.

My diagnosis was hardest on Samantha, but she determined her role from the start - caregiver. Mack was younger and couldn't truly grasp what cancer meant. He was primarily concerned with what was going to happen to my hair. I didn't look sick. I didn't act too sick. He saw how tired I was after I started chemo. He saw me lay in the bathroom floor on a blanket near the toilet. He watched me and hugged me. He carried around hand sanitizer all the time. If I touched anything he said, "Hold out your hand, Ma. You gotta get rid of those germs." He didn't let me open the doors or push the grocery cart. Too many germs.

"Remember Mama; the doctor said you have to be careful about germs now."

When my hair fell out, Samantha hugged me and held me. Mack was afraid of me. When I was bald, I looked sick.

My kids loved the stories I made up for them when they were growing up. Their favorite was a story about Aubrey, a mischievous albino bat and Ghostly, a little boy ghost. Each night the three of us would lie on one of their beds and I would tell them Ghosty and Aubrey's latest exploits. A few days after I lost my hair, I told them that Aubrey snuck into Mack's backpack and had gone to school with him. She spent the entire day getting him into trouble. Samantha and Mack laughed.

"Tell us more," they begged.

As I continued with the adventures of Aubrey, I noticed Mack was rubbing my head. He hadn't really touched me or hugged me since my hair fell out. I think he noticed he was rubbing my bald head about the same time I did.

He looked at me and grinned. "Your head feels cool, Ma. I love you".

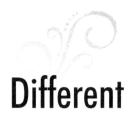

Different

I never wanted to be Cancer Cathleen. I didn't want to be different in that way. People change how they act around you when you are diagnosed. They don't mean to. They just don't know how to act; do they say something, or do they ignore your cancer diagnosis. They feel awkward and that makes you feel self-conscious.

I set out on an unintentional mission to make sure I didn't appear different. I started with the cancer center. There were incredible people working at the Southwest Cancer Center in Lubbock, Texas. I could only imagine the amount of stress they went through each day. I wanted to give back to the people that were helping me. As a thank you, I began offering yoga classes to the staff of the cancer center. Looking back, I believe I wanted to help them, but I also wanted them to see me and know me. I didn't want to be just another breast cancer patient.

When I was diagnosed with cancer I was:

- Working as the Executive Coordinator to the CEO of a company 20 hours a week
- Teaching 5-8 fitness classes a week
- Preparing to test for my black belt in Tae Kwon Do
- A fundraising Chairman for a volunteer organization
- The mother of a 6th and 10th grader
- The wife of a recently retired Army Lieutenant Colonel who had just started a small business

I was busy. I was too busy for cancer. Cancer demanded that I slow down. I said, "Hell No"! And pushed even harder. I worked so hard to maintain the life I had before cancer. What I didn't realize then was that I couldn't hide from it. I could continue to discount the reality of cancer but that doesn't lessen the fear. I could tell everyone I knew I was going to beat it. I made it my job to show that cancer wasn't that bad. It didn't matter how many times I said it, I never believed it.

I tried to hide under a wig. Wigs were uncomfortable and itchy, but they gave me a place to hide. I wore a wig anytime I went out of the house. If I didn't, people might look at me and feel pity. I wanted to blend in - not stick out. People would whisper, "Have you heard Cathleen Reid has cancer?" It wasn't meant to be mean. It was just news. I could not stomach anyone pitying me. The people who knew me didn't pity me. They loved me and wanted me to be ok.

There are numerous options when you walk up to someone that has cancer. I heard them all.

- "I am soooooo sorry. I heard you have cancer."
- "How are you?" – said in a very sad and pitying tone.
- "Tell me all about it. What stage are you? Did they get it all? Do you have to have chemo?"
- "You know my grandmother/mother/aunt/neighbor had breast cancer. She sure was a fighter. She died about six months after diagnosis, but I remember how strong she was."
- "I am so sorry; how long do you have?"
- "Well, I guess you'll lose all that pretty hair of yours, then you'll know how the rest of us feel."

They wanted to make me feel better but how they often came out, it rarely did

When people talk about cancer survivors it used to annoy me. I felt pitied. What I didn't realize was that they were recognizing how hard it was, that we cancer survivors have gone through something difficult and survived. I still don't like pity, I never will. I saw the concern as pity. From now on, I am going to see it as recognition. Recognition that I am a warrior – a survivor.

Radiation & Tattoos - a poem

I never thought I would get a tattoo.
Not two ugly black dots; one between my breasts and one under my arm.
I didn't know radiology technicians did tattoos.
I didn't know, until that first appointment, that I was getting a tattoo.
"You have to be here every day for radiation – for seven weeks. The tattoo helps us with placement".

Radiation.
Put a gown on.
Leave it open in the front.
Lay on the table.
The machine is above me.
Light goes on.
There is a grid on my chest.
They center the grid over the area to be radiated.

It didn't take long -- ten minutes? I don't remember.
It wasn't hard.
I had a false sense of relief that first day.
Each time I went to radiation they seemed to drain more of my energy and strength.
I went to radiation alone.
I didn't need anyone to go with me.
The girls in the radiation clinic became by yoga friends.

Red.
Raw.

Sick.
Pain.
Tired.
Anxiety.

Every week I had an appointment with the radiation oncologist to see
how I was doing.
He was so impressed with how well I was handling radiation. Most
people didn't handle it as well.
I was strong.
It can't beat me.

Day 20 of 35

My chest hurts.
The area over my incision is broken open and raw.
I'm tired but I can't sleep.
I am still teaching aerobics and working.
I can't breathe.
Don't make me go.
Mom, I hurt.
Mom, I need someone to hold me.
I need someone who will give me some of their strength – mine is all
used up.

I'm empty.

Waiting for the doctor.
There is not enough air in the room.
Why am I crying?
The doctor walks in.
I'm crying.
I'm shaking.
I need air.
He looks worried.

I know he is wondering what I did with the incredibly strong woman
he saw last week.
The woman last week was tired, but she was a fighter.

This woman…
This woman who is sitting on the exam table
in that gown is crumbling before his eyes.
The doctor is pleasant but sterile. He isn't as warm and fuzzy as my
oncologist.
I am so embarrassed.
I am letting him down.
He was so proud of my strength.
      Maybe he was planning on giving me the Radiation Medal of
Valor.

He doesn't know what to do and I can't help him.
I'm drowning.
I need help.
Make this pain stop.
I need sleep.
I have an open seeping wound
In pain
Tired
But I can't close my eyes.

The room is getting smaller.
I need someone to lean on.
I need
      I need
            I need
This to be over.

He prescribes an anti-anxiety medication
      or maybe it is an anti-depressant or
      a sleeping pills.

He throws everything he can think of at me.

I was at the bottom on day 20.

When I paused…
When I slowed my mind down…
    I looked up.
    There was light.
    There was air.

Day 20
    A glimmer of the end was in sight.
Day 20
    I was more than ½ way through.
Day 20
    I hurt.
    I was so tired.
    I needed …
        What? I don't really know.

I needed something or someone to help me make it to-day 35.
I was starting to get a little fuzz on my head, but I was still bald.
Bald
Raw
and
Tired.

Was I falling apart because it was day 20 or had I just used up all my strength?

My strength;
    They could have written a ballad to my strength.
    If they could have bottled my strength….

The radiation technician said they could fill in the tattoo with a flesh color after I was done.
I think I'll keep it.

It is ugly like this time in my life.
It is a black blob or maybe it is a starting point.

To remember.
To remember when I am at the bottom to look up.

Yoga for Stress, Anxiety, Depression

Radiation was hard. Radiation took all of my energy. I had been counting on that energy to get me through the treatment. I was left raw and tired. Yoga can help lower your anxiety, depression and stress.

I had a yoga practice in place and it helped tremendously. It did not keep me from feeling tired, stressed, anxiety-laden and raw but it made the side effects easier. I had to be more careful of the poses during this time. I had burns, open sores and aches that I had to work around.

I felt little peace during chemotherapy, but I felt even less during radiation treatment.

Affirmation: I am peace.

Poses:
You can do these individually or put them into a flow together.

Mountain Pose
Reach up to the sky
Chair
Fold down to a Forward Fold
Step back the right foot back to a Low Crescent Lunge – hands on the floor, left leg in front
Plank
Downward Facing Dog

Step forward with the left leg into Warrior II
Crescent lunge
Step into Mountain Pose and do other side.
Flow through these poses as long as it feels good to you.
Move to Seated Forward Fold
Cow Face Pose
Seated Straddle
Reclined Bound Angle
Savasana

Mountain pose was grounding and helped me to feel present. Chair pose, like plank pose and downward facing dog pose reminded me that I am strong. The emotional release of forward fold, the hip opening in Warrior II and the balancing aspect of crescent lunge all helped me stay strong. Seated forward fold stretches the back and hamstrings. Seated straddle pose, and reclined bound angle help to relax and lessen stress.

Doing this flow during radiation will be easier at the beginning of the treatment. As you get further into the treatment, you may find you are uncomfortable with some of the arm movements, modify to make it work for you.

Yoga for Stress,

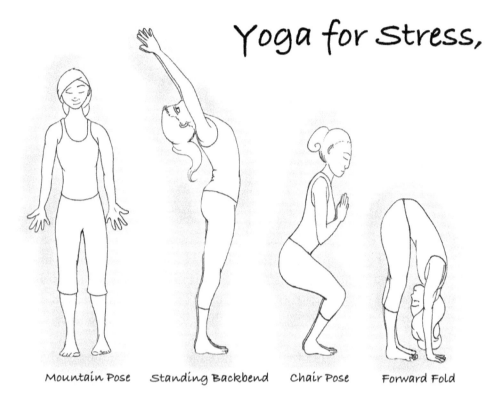

Mountain Pose   Standing Backbend   Chair Pose   Forward Fold

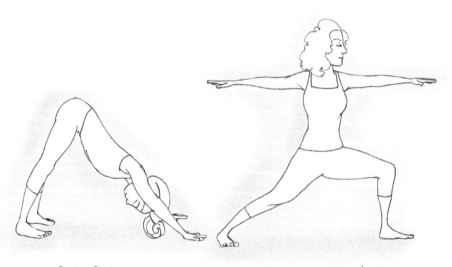

Down Dog   Warrior II

Anxiety, and Depression

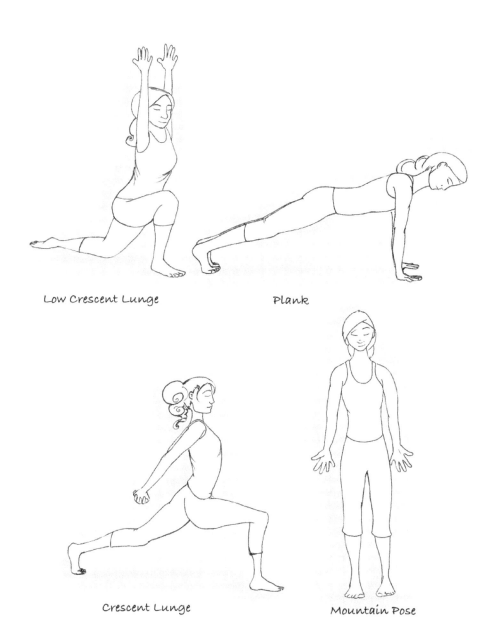

Low Crescent Lunge

Plank

Crescent Lunge

Mountain Pose

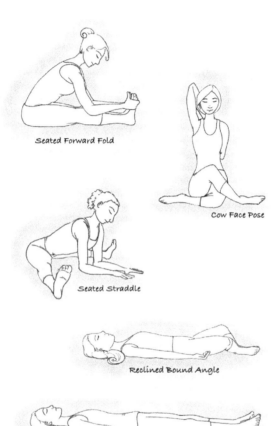

Seated Forward Fold

Cow Face Pose

Seated Straddle

Reclined Bound Angle

Savasana

Red M & M's

I hate "why me". I hate pity parties, though I have been known to have them. Nothing good can come out of feeling sorry for yourself. You can't make things better by curling up in a ball and crying why me all the time.

When I was diagnosed with breast cancer, I cried. I was scared. I asked why me. We all know we are going to die. No one wants to know what the instrument of their death will be or when they will die. I suppose if we knew that we might live completely different lives. If we lived different lives would that change how we died and what killed us? I can ramble on about that for days. My diagnosis brought me face to face with the reality that I would not live forever. I am mortal.

Why did I get breast cancer? What caused it? Why did it happen to me? I worked out, I ate a healthy diet. What did I do wrong? Was it because I used spray deodorant when I was young? Was it the hormones in the meat? The hair color I used? Was it red M&M's? Was it the stress of a struggling marriage? I remember smelling the gas fumes when I was young as my Dad filled the car with fuel, could that have been it? Did I not eat enough fiber? Too much fiber? Too much coffee? Should I have banned all sugar from my diet? Was it the year I tried to smoke cigarettes in college? Do I wear too much black? Was my faith not strong enough? Should I have prayed more? Or was it just something that randomly that happened?

No one ever wants to think cancer will happen to them. They think cancer will bypass them, bypass their use of cigarettes, alcohol, tanning beds, the fast food they eat and the stress they carry. I have heard smokers say, "well, *something* is gonna kill me". We know some things are bad for us, but we never believe we will get cancer.

I will never know why I got cancer. I have decided it was the amount of stress I was dealing with at the time. The oncologist said they don't know why I got cancer, but he did ask if I was dealing with a large amount of stress.

I got cancer. I don't know why. I refused to let cancer define me and how I would live my life. I spent many years existing in a life that was happening around me. I knew many people that saw cancer as a wake-up call. It was a cold, harsh wake-up call but I am thankful for the realization that I wasn't living before cancer. I was just existing.

I am living now and will live and appreciate each second, I have, each breath I take, and the people that surround me. Why me? Why not me?

Yoga for Joy

I want to consider myself a joyful person. I am most of the time. I often felt sorry for myself when I was going through breast cancer. Try this flow when you are feeling sad. Repeat each piece of the flow as long as it feels good to you. This flow can give you a release, a feeling of freedom and joy.

Affirmation: I am joyful

Poses:
Mountain Pose
Stretch up to the sky
Grab your right wrist with your left hand and stretch your body to the left
Grab your left wrist with your right hand and stretch your body to the right
Standing backbend – listen to your body.
Repeat

Forward Fold
Downward Facing Dog
Upward Facing Dog
Forward Fold
Repeat 8 times

Flowing ½ camel (extended Childs pose, slide left hand back to left heel, ½ Camel – other side)

Repeat 4-8 times, taking your time and breath. Noticing how your feel. Feel your body. You are alive.

Move to Downward Facing Dog
Lunge forward to Crescent Lunge and clasp hand behind your back (keep elbows bent or straighten) Open to Sun God. Back to Crescent Lunge. Downward Facing Dog.
Repeat other side.

Reclined Bound Angle
Knees to Chest
Lying Spinal Twist each side

When you have finished the flow, lie down on your mat for relaxation. Savasana is not nap time though I do have students that have fallen asleep. The intent is to stay alert but relaxed. This is hard for many students but is helpful to everyone, especially for cancer patients. I like to have my students open their palms to the ceiling and let their legs flop out. As you lie in relaxation pose allow your muscles to release. This is a time for you, don't cheat yourself out of this part of your practice.

Yoga Practice Notes

Yoga For Joy

Flow A

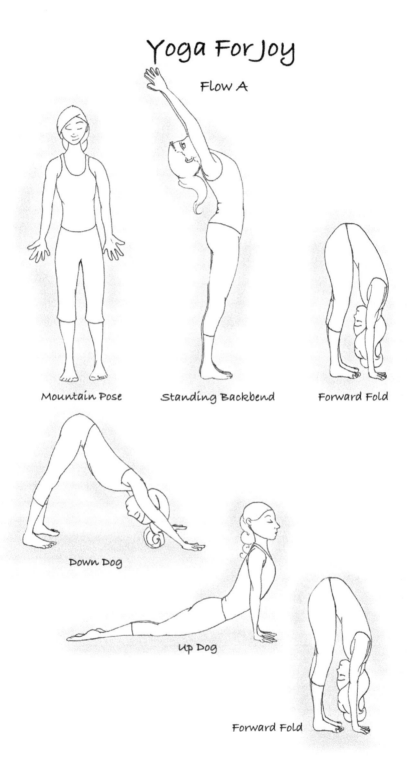

Mountain Pose

Standing Backbend

Forward Fold

Down Dog

Up Dog

Forward Fold

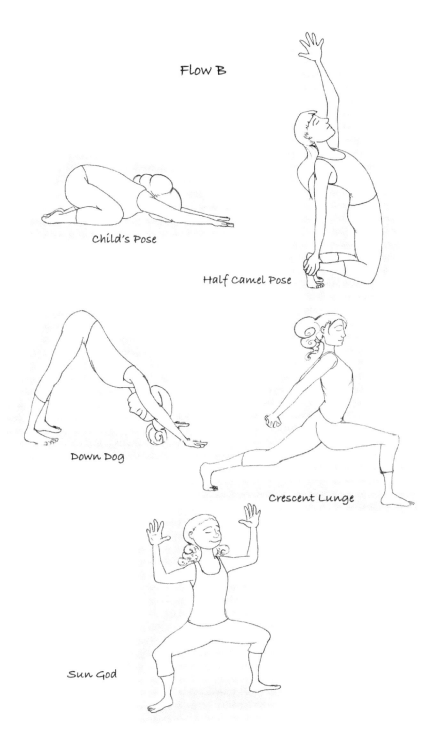

Flow B

Child's Pose

Half Camel Pose

Down Dog

Crescent Lunge

Sun God

Yoga for Joy Continued

Flow C

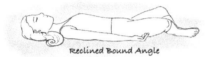
Reclined Bound Angle

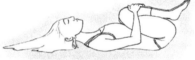
Knees to Chest

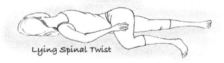
Lying Spinal Twist

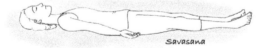
Savasana

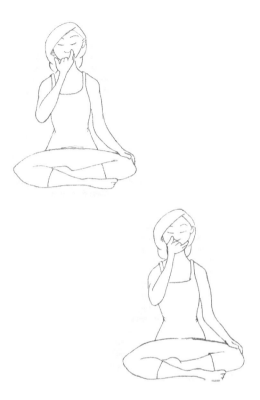

Alternate Nostril Breathing

We use nose breathing in yoga. We breath this way so the air is warmed and filtered as it enters our body. Breathing through your nose also requires more concentration which helps you stay focused.

Alternate nostril breathing is a breathing technique that is used during meditation or toward the end of class as a way to cool down. I will often use it at the beginning to help the class calm and focus their minds. My evening classes are often filled with people rushing in from work and this breath is a nice way to deliberately slow them down.

- Take your right hand and tuck your third and index finger in towards your palm. Place your fourth finger on your left nostril with your thumb on your right nostril. Close off your right nostril with your thumb and inhale through your left. Close your left with your fourth finger and exhale evenly through your right. Inhale through your right again. At the top of the breath, close the right and exhale through the left.

Alternate nostril breathing: calms the mind, lowers heart rate, soothes headaches and helps to adjust perspective.

Savage Mask

"You are such a positive person. Everyone is drawn to your positive energy. You have already helped several patients that have wanted to talk to you. You would be a great help to others. You have handled the treatments and side effects so well."

Dr. Cobos wanted me to go to a cancer support group.

I should have gone. I always tried to give back to others, but I couldn't be around negativity. I was barely holding on. I was using all the strength I had to keep the façade of strength in place. Dr. Cobos was amazed at my strength. I never considered myself an actress, but I was an award-winning actress on this stage.

Everyone was proud and amazed at how I remained positive and strong. I didn't have another option. I don't remember there being another option. Be strong or curl into the fetal position and cry. No choice in my mind. Negativity and self-pity kill. They eat all your reserves of hope for dinner.

I wore my strength like a badge of honor and this badge protected me. I was so strong that some people forgot I was going through chemo. It was easy for them to forget when I was running around in my Super Hero Wig pretending to have loads of energy. I was so strong that even some people in my family forgot. I was so strong, I was invincible. Yeah, right.

I look back now at why I didn't want to go to a cancer support group. The people scared me. I asked if it was a place that people cried and felt sorry for themselves.

"Sometimes," said Dr. Cobos.

I could have gone, just to see if it was a group that understood the fear I was hiding. I was afraid they would see right through me and shatter this fragile mask I was wearing. The mask I had so savagely built. I built my strength with anger. Why did I get cancer? It is not fair. I did everything right. Now I am a member of the Cancer Club, a lifetime member.

Now the doctor and nurses wanted me to go - with my fear, my anxiety, my anger – and help someone else by giving them all the hope I had left. I couldn't.

I remember making that decision. I regret making that decision. I should have gone. If I had shared my hope, maybe more hope would have grown in my heart. I won't ever know that now. I didn't realize how much it hurt my soul when I didn't try to help more people during that time of my life. The cancer patients that reached out to me were better prepared for what was to come because of my words – they told me that later.

If there is one person that reads my words now and is affected positively, one person that I can help because of the experiences I have had then it's not too late. That's why I keep writing.

Yoga for Courage

You need courage to get through diagnosis, treatment and recovery from breast cancer treatments. I love the chest opening and back bending aspects of sun salute C. Moving from child's pose to ½ camel you feel the release of child's pose and the heart opening of camel. Try this flow when you need a shot of courage.

Affirmation: I am courageous

Poses:

Sun Salute C,
Mountain pose, reach up standing backbend
Forward fold
Crescent Lunge, right leg in front
Plank
Upward Facing Dog
Downward Facing Dog
Crescent Lunge, left leg in front
Forward Fold
Standing Backbend back to Mountain Pose

Sun Salute C, repeat 2 times with a low lunge
Sun Salute C, repeat 4 times with a crescent lunge
Mountain Pose – say to yourself I am, on the inhale and courageous, on the exhale.

Move to child's pose with arms extended out in front

Slide left arm back to left heel as you come up to ½ camel pose
Move back to extended child's pose
Slide right arm back to right heel as you come up to ½ camel pose
Repeat this flow slowly, 2-8 times on each side

Move to a wide legged child's pose with your forehead on your two fists and breath.
Breath in, I am and exhale, courageous.

Yoga Practice Notes

Yoga for Courage

Sun Salute C

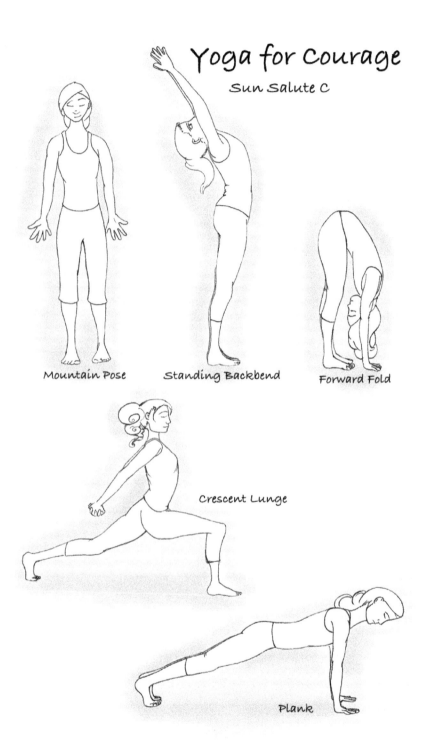

Mountain Pose

Standing Backbend

Forward Fold

Crescent Lunge

Plank

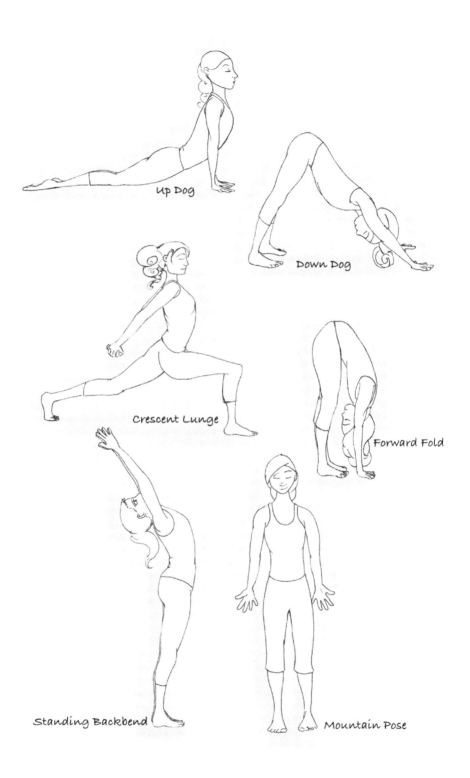

Up Dog

Down Dog

Crescent Lunge

Forward Fold

Standing Backbend

Mountain Pose

Yoga for Courage Continued

Heart Opening Flow

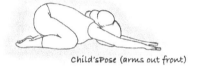

Child'sPose (arms out front)

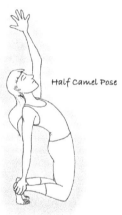

Half Camel Pose

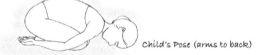

Child's Pose (arms to back)

Positive Affirmations

Have you ever felt sad and didn't know why? Have you ever cried for no reason at all?

I started saying positive affirmations to myself when I was going through chemotherapy. I didn't feel like any of the things that I said to myself in the mirror were true. That is why I had to say them.

When I was going through treatments for breast cancer, I was scared, and I was furious at my body for betraying me. I would look in the mirror in disgust each morning as I tried to put on my makeup. No one told me how hard it was to put on makeup during chemotherapy. I had to have all clean applicators each day. My foundation went on just like normal, but the rest was a challenge. I could not use my blush brush, so my blush went onto my cheeks in streaks with a cotton ball. It is difficult to put eye shadow on with a Q-tip, but I needed something disposable. I had a client that sold Mary Kay makeup and she brought me mascara wands, so I could throw them away after each application. It was frustrating. I had gone to an information event at the cancer center and had been given some new products to try since I couldn't use my own that had been opened.

Each morning after my shower, I would walk to the mirror and begin. I was not very nice to myself. My skin was dull, and I had gained weight. I always felt nauseous and tired and scared. My eyes no longer sparkled. I didn't realize I was saying negative things about myself as I put on my makeup each day.

I am mad.

I hate the way I look.
I am fat.
Why doesn't David love me?
I am unloved.

Stop it! I am lucky they caught my cancer early. My kids love me. I am loved. But . . .

My body is tired.
I am hurting.
I am bald.
My skin is dull.
I am stupid to have let this happen to me.

One day, as I went through the list of things that were wrong with me, I just stopped. I started replacing the negatives with positives. If I said something negative to myself I would immediately stop and change it to a positive. I didn't believe it, but I wanted to believe it. The hardest ones to say, the ones that made me cry were, "I am strong. I am intelligent. I am beautiful." I didn't believe them at all, but I desperately wanted to.

I am strong.
I am free.
I am healed.
I am whole.
I am loved.
I am beautiful.

Then why do I feel so bad?

I am happy.
I am deserving.
I am calm.
I am fulfilled.
I am successful.
I am going to get better.

Then why does it feel like I will never feel joy again?

It was hard for me to stand in front of the mirror and tell myself the things that I wanted to believe. It's hard to be positive when you're fighting cancer. I have always been happy, but it's tough to maintain a positive spin when you are dealing with a cancer diagnosis. And yet, I had to believe I would be healthy again.

I wrote out a list of over twenty positive affirmations and I posted them on the counter in the bathroom. I looked at the list. I looked at myself. The list. Me.

My skin did not have a healthy glow. My eyes looked glazed. I had to look hard to see the me that was there before chemo. As I read my list aloud they sounded hollow but reading them made me stand up straighter. I wanted the words to be true so much that I started to believe them. I read my positive affirmations each day. Some days I read them crying. Some days I read them with doubt. Eventually my desire for them to become my personal truth took hold.

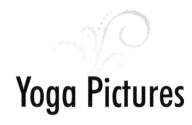

Yoga Pictures

I love to take pictures of my yoga students in poses. Most of my students know why I take pictures, but I think they sometimes forget the reason because they have fun participating in my ideas.

I teach yoga for all the reasons that most yoga instructors teach yoga:

- To help make a difference in someone else's life
- To help people recover from injury, be healthier, be more fit, increase flexibility
- To connect with others

I take pictures of my yogi's because I want them to see themselves the same way I see them. Beautiful.

My evening classes are filled with people that have worked hard all day – in an office, a school, traveling, as a parent, a teacher, in the medical profession, a factory and many other jobs. One evening one of my regulars was in class. She had been coming to class for a few months and her backbends had improved significantly. She loves backbends and has a naturally flexible back.

I don't like having mirrors in the class but sometimes I like to show people how they look in a pose. I take pictures with my iPhone to show people their progress. That night we worked on backbending poses and this student's backbend was beautiful.

"Can I take a picture of your backbend, so you can see how gorgeous it is?" I asked.

"I don't like pictures of myself"

"I will delete it immediately," I told her. "I only want to show you how graceful you look in this pose."

"Ok," she said, "but you promise you'll delete it immediately?"

"Yes, ma'am."

She moved into her backbend. I snapped her picture and showed it to her. She stared at it is disbelief for a moment. "I'm beautiful," she said. "Can you send me that picture, so I can show my husband?" she asked with a smile.

A few weeks later, another yogi who usually avoided pictures came to class. I had shown her earlier how she had been progressing in a pose. This woman was on the road traveling for work each day. She had a young child and loads of stress. She walked into class, rolled out her mat, looked me in the eye and said, "Make me feel pretty."

I love to take pictures of my yogi's. I love to show them their progress but more than that, I want them to see for themselves how beautiful they are.

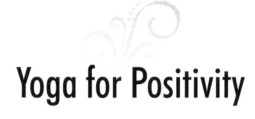

Yoga for Positivity

I didn't always stay positive during treatments for cancer. I am not always positive today. I try to be aware when negativity starts creeping in. I chose the poses in this flow because of the hip opening and energizing benefits of these poses. These poses make me feel better and generally make me less stressed. They help to increase my happiness. Positivity can help to combat negativity.

Affirmation: I am optimistic

Poses:

Sun god to temple, back to sun god then to temple.
Flow to each side 8 times

Add:
Crescent lunge
Warrior I
Tree
Warrior II
Back to Sun God and do the other side

Yoga Practice Notes

Yoga for Positivity

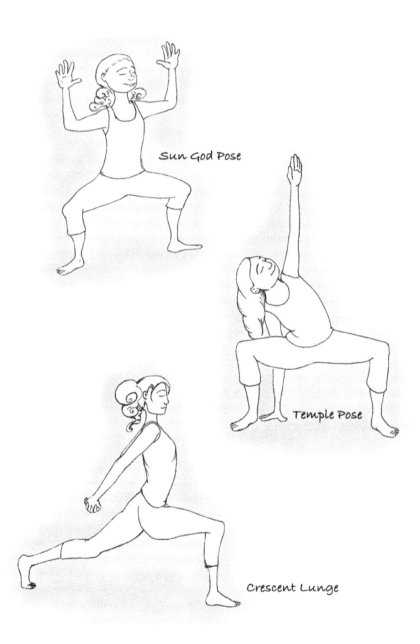

Sun God Pose

Temple Pose

Crescent Lunge

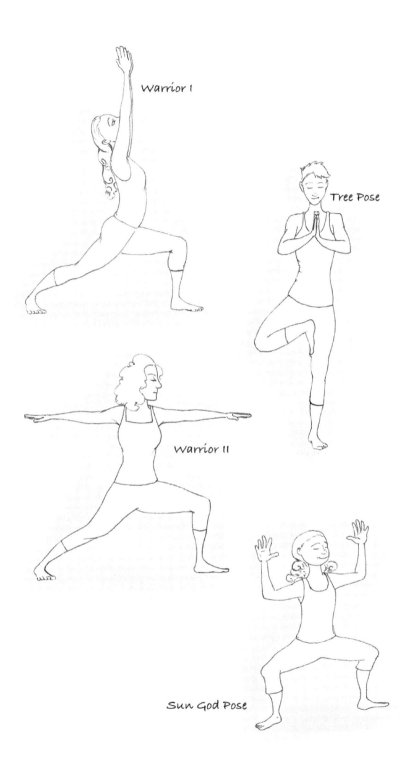

Warrior I

Tree Pose

Warrior II

Sun God Pose

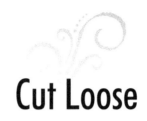

Cut Loose

When I was going through treatments, I had my blood drawn weekly. The doctors were checking my white blood cell count constantly. After chemo was finished, I still went in regularly to get my blood drawn.

Weekly.
Bi-weekly.
Monthly.
Every three months.
Every six months.
Once a year with my mammogram.

I experienced fear each year when I went to see my oncologist but the visit had become my security blanket. I began seeing Dr. Davidson when I moved to Tennessee in 2009. Dr. Davidson had my back.

Cancer had been a part of my life since November 13, 2006. It will always be a part of me. Cancer does not define who I am but cancer changed me. I look for the positives in all situations. When I was diagnosed with breast cancer, I did not look for positives. As I moved through treatment, I had to be positive.

Each time the doctor told me I didn't have to come back for a longer period, I should have felt joy. I didn't. I should have felt relief that I was healed. I didn't. Was I cured? Do you really ever say you are cured of cancer? There is no cure, so what do you say? Every time the distance between appointments was lengthened, I was scared. What if they thought they got it all but they didn't? What if I came back in three months and it was too late?

I thought about the "what if's" frequently during treatment and the first few years after I finished chemotherapy and radiation. I saw my oncologist for yearly check-ups and five years after my treatments ended, he told me he could cut me loose. I didn't need to see him anymore. My BRAC genetic test for breast cancer was negative. The results of my oncotype test showed less than a 1% chance of recurrence. He felt comfortable not seeing me anymore.

I sat. I didn't breathe or blink. I felt sick to my stomach. It was irrational, but I felt the same fear I felt when I was initially diagnosed. He watched as I processed what he told me. I didn't speak.

I looked at Dr. Davidson. I wanted to be positive my cancer was gone. I was positive I wasn't ready to be set free. He smiled at me and said he would see me in a year. Maybe then, I'd be ready to be cut loose.

Sisterhood of Survivors

As I was getting ready to teach a beginner yoga class, a beautiful woman came in to take a class with her daughter and mother. Have you ever met someone and felt an immediate connection to him or her? I knew this woman was a breast cancer survivor because I had spoken to her mother, one of my students, about her. I knew immediately this woman understood what I had been through and I knew what she had been through. We didn't have to say a word.

There is a peculiar bond when meeting someone who has gone through what you have gone through. It is comforting to meet someone that understands what you can't say out loud. That can happen by going to the same school, growing up in the same town, finding out you both like horses or have the same hobbies. I've found it interesting that there is a whole sisterhood of breast cancer patients, survivors, and the people in their lives that have been affected by breast cancer. Cancer creates a link.

I found that out when I was initially diagnosed with breast cancer. People started coming out of the woodwork letting me know that they knew someone who had faced the disease. Acquaintances shared with me that they were survivors. It was surprising how many people were touched in some way by breast cancer. It made me uncomfortable, yet at the same time it was reassuring.

When I moved to Tennessee, there was a lady I worked with that was a breast cancer survivor. She had been cancer free for over 20 years. When she found out I had been through breast cancer, she said we were sisters. She said we had both gone through something hard and survived. She said cancer sucked but cancer couldn't beat us. It was oddly soothing to have her be so blunt with me. I have been told often about women who lost their battle with breast cancer. I am always scared for myself when I hear a story of a friend/mother/sister who died after a reoccurrence of breast cancer. It feels like people love to share these stories more often than survivor stories. I suppose they want to share the memory of someone they loved with me.

I used to keep my breast cancer story to myself. I don't now. People want to connect with someone who is a survivor. Women who have gone through breast cancer can't express to others how it feels. It is hard to convey to someone else how it feels to have a part of your femininity turn against you. They know the nausea of chemotherapy and the burning of radiation. They know how it feels to look mortality in the eye. Breast cancer survivors don't' have to tell each other how it felt to go through it, they know. The connection is unspoken.

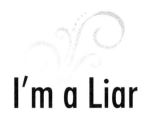

I'm a Liar

Have you ever wondered about the lies you tell yourself? We tell ourselves lies for so long that they become truths. Sometimes we desire an outcome so badly that we make it truth just to fit the narrative. Or maybe we doubt ourselves so much that a lie becomes a reality.

What are my truths? What are my lies?

I am a positive person. Is this a truth or a lie? This is a truth. I am positive. I see the best in life. This can also be one of my lies. I desperately need to see the positive so much so that I often paint negatives to make them positive.

I am a happy person. That is a truth. I have down days like everyone, but I don't like people to see that part of me. I need to be seen by the outside world as happy all the time. Why? So, I will be liked and accepted? If I admit I am not happy all the time, who will like or love me? The rational woman within me knows that people love me for who I am. I took to heart the admonition as a little girl that I should always keep a smile on my face.

I am caring. I care about the people around me. I love and care for my family. This is a truth.

I had cancer and handled it with strength and a positive attitude. This is truth. The part of my breast cancer story that is a big, fat lie is telling people that it was not a big deal, telling people that I was lucky to have only had breast cancer and not a disease I would have to live with the rest of my life. My cancer was going to be defeated but people with Multiple Sclerosis, Diabetes, Lupus or Parkinson's Disease were not as lucky.

I maintained my perky attitude about my diagnosis because I didn't want to face the reality of cancer. The truth in my cancer journey is that I am now a stronger and more confident person because of it.

I am a coward. This was a truth before I had cancer. I do not like confrontation and will avoid it at almost any cost. I don't know why I got breast cancer, but I do know that the stress in my marriage during that time did not help my health.

I was a good and trusting wife. This is a truth and a lie. I was an encouraging and supportive wife. I supported my military husband through all our moves, the deployments, the new jobs, all the required activities and the new locations where we were stationed. I kept a clean, organized and attractive home. I entertained. The lie came when I no longer loved him.

I am able to be focused with my thoughts. You would think this is a truth since I am a yogi. It is difficult for me to be still. I used to believe it was because I was an active person. When I am still, I have time to think and center. Being still is when I am the most creative, but it is also when I have time to think about challenges. I have stayed in motion to keep from doing this.

I am beautiful. That is always a hard affirmation for me to say. Does it make me conceited to say I am beautiful? I suppose it would if I believed my outer looks defined who I am. I believe I am beautiful because I see beauty in others.

I am loved. This is so very true. There are so many people that love and care about me. The lie in this is the fact that I did not love myself for a very long time. It has been a journey to get to a place where I love myself. I love the woman I am now. That is a truth.

I Wonder — a poem

I wonder what I will be doing in a year from now.
Will I be happy?
I wonder what color my hair would be if I didn't color it. When will it snow again?
Can dogs understand what we say? Can I run a marathon? Am I a good person?
I wonder if I can be forgiven.
I wonder if I will finish my book. Why does the smell of cinnamon make me happy?
I wonder if anyone, besides my children, will ever appreciate my sense of humor.
Is there anyone who would love me as I am?
Why don't people feel the magic of Christmas anymore? Will I ever own a horse again?
I wonder if there is life on other planets. Will I always have to make the coffee?

> I wonder if God loves all of us, no matter what we believe and what we do.

How did I get so lucky to have such wonderful children? Will I be alone for the rest of my life?
Would I rather be alone than with someone that doesn't love me? Why are my toes always cold?
I wonder if I will be remembered.
How was I blessed with so many great friends? Can I be loved. Will I ever see Scotland?
Does anyone else sit around and wonder random things?

Am I weird?
I wonder why I got cancer.
I wonder if I will ever feel safe again.
I wonder if I will always wonder.

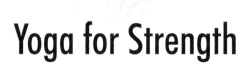

Yoga for Strength

When I began teaching yoga I often heard, "isn't yoga just stretching?". New students were always surprised to find out that yoga could be challenging. It is important to maintain strong bodies. It was especially important to me during cancer treatment. I read that the treatments could cause bone loss, so I wanted to do everything I could to stay strong. This flow is full of strength building poses and should be done at your own pace. The repetitions and times that I have included are suggestions. Remember you should always listen to your own body and work when you need to be each day.

Affirmation: I am strong

Poses:

Warm-up, Sun Salute A, repeat 3-8 times

Plank – full or modified, 30-60 seconds

Side Plank – full or modified, 10 seconds each side

Downward Facing Dog, to rest and reset breath

Dolphin, 30 seconds

Forearm Plank, 30-60 seconds

Forearms Side Plank, 10 seconds each side

Childs pose to reset breath

Repeat entire flow, 1 – 5 times

Yoga for Strength

Sun Salute A

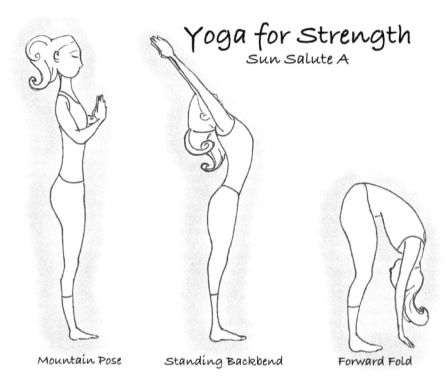

Mountain Pose   Standing Backbend   Forward Fold

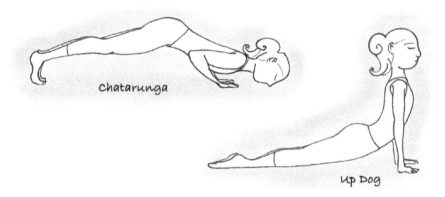

Chatarunga   Up Dog

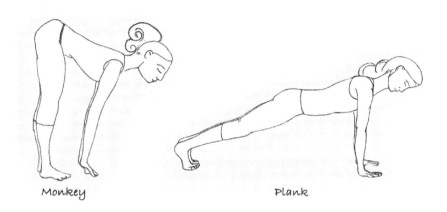

Monkey

Plank

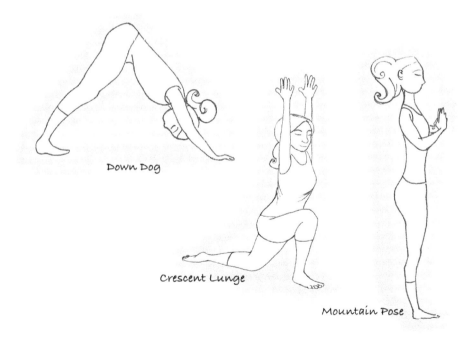

Down Dog

Crescent Lunge

Mountain Pose

Strength Holds

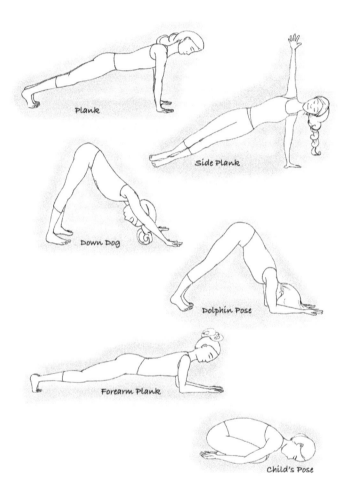

Plank

Side Plank

Down Dog

Dolphin Pose

Forearm Plank

Child's Pose

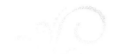

Heartache

I just read a strong and terribly sad blog post written by a daughter about the recurrence of her mother's cancer. Recurrence is a fear all cancer patients live with forever. I am ten years' cancer free and I still stress out when it is time for my visit to the oncologist. I usually see my oncologist in November each year. In October I become aware again that I am a cancer survivor. How can a breast cancer survivor/patient miss it with all the pink ribbons adorning everything? I remember getting so many items covered with pink ribbons when I was diagnosed. I was even given pink yoga pants. Pink was my least favorite color and my life was quickly accented with pink. October is a hard month for me because of the reminders that are everywhere. November brings stress as I wait to get the results of my tumor markers. I am always glad I go in a week early to get my blood drawn so I can get the results from my oncologist. The week between the blood draw and my appointment is hard. I replay scenarios in my head. I worry. I stress. I pray. After I see my oncologist and get a clean bill of health I only get a short reprieve. My mammogram is usually in December.

I get the reminder in October. I feel the stress in November. The fear arrives in December. It is not normal fear like you feel when you see a scary movie or see a snake or fear rejection, failure or heights. It is a fear that hits you in the pit of your stomach. It is an indescribable fear that cancer patients know well. It is fear of having to go through chemo again, of losing your hair again, of radiation, of nausea, of exhaustion. It is the fear of death.

I never like reading or hearing about recurrence. Recurrence shouldn't happen. Recurrence is always in the back of cancer patient's minds, even when they have had all the tests that tell them there is a low chance the cancer will return.

I am always surprised that people want to share with me that they have a loved one whose cancer returned. Hearing that always evokes fear.

I cannot think of any words to say to ease the anger and fear this daughter felt for her mother. I am at a loss and that does not happen to me often. I feel as though I cannot read something so raw and not comment. There is nothing to say to make this daughter feel better. My heart aches for her and for her mother.

The Waiting Room - a poem

Last night before my appointment, the fear was there.
It's that time of the year.
Time to go see the oncologist.
I am fine.
I know I am fine.
That knowledge doesn't ease the fear.
Today.
It's 3:00pm.
I'm sitting in the waiting room.
My appointment isn't until 3:30pm
but I'm early.
I'm always
early.
I get here early so maybe they will call me back sooner.
Then I'll know I'm fine sooner.
It's 3:15pm.
I am still sitting in the waiting room.
My pulse is beating hard enough for me to notice.
The anxiety has stepped up to be noticed.
I have sweat on my upper lip.
I cross and uncross my legs.
3:25pm.
Sitting in the waiting room.
I have already flipped through all the old Redbook, Good Housekeeping,
and Better Homes and Gardens magazines on the coffee table.
I need to go to the bathroom.
They will weigh me – I must go to the bathroom.

3:30pm.

It's time.

Why haven't they called me?

I came in before him.

Why does he get to go back before me?

Should I check to make sure they remember I'm here?

3:45pm.

I check the email on my phone.

I send text messages to anyone I think might message me back.

I start reading a boring book for work.

I can't focus.

I bite my nails.

How did my heart get in my throat?

I am watching the receptionist.

If I make eye contact

she will have to call me back.

3:50pm.

Cathleen Reid?

It's time.

The Cooling Breath (Sitali/Sitkari)

Sitali breath is often translated as "the cooling breath" because the act of breathing in the air across the tongue and into the mouth can have a cooling and calming effect.

To practice Sitali, you need to be able to curl the sides of your tongue inward so that it looks like a straw. The ability to curl the tongue is a genetic trait. If you can't, try an alternative technique called Sitkari which offers the same effects. Sitali and Sitkari breathing techniques are a great way to energize you.

Sitali breathing:

Sit comfortably, either in a chair or on the floor, with your shoulders relaxed and your spine naturally erect. Slightly lower the chin, curl the tongue lengthwise, and project it out of the mouth to a comfortable distance. Inhale gently through the "straw" formed by your curled tongue as you slowly lift your chin toward the ceiling, lifting only as far as the neck is comfortable. At the end of the inhalation, with your chin comfortably raised, retract the tongue and close the mouth. Exhale slowly through the nostrils as you gently lower your chin back to a neutral position. Repeat for 8 to 12 breaths.

Sitkari breathing:

Open the mouth slightly with your tongue just behind the teeth. Inhale slowly through the space between the upper and lower teeth, letting the air move into your body as you raise your chin slightly. At the end of the inhalation, close the mouth and exhale through the nostrils as you slowly lower your chin back to neutral. Repeat for 8 to 12 breaths.

Each time I teach this technique in class to children, and some adults, it causes them to smile. It feels good. This breath can help to reduce anger, energize you and lessen anxiety.

I Am Different Now

After my diagnosis
the mammogram
the biopsy
the lumpectomy
the surgery for the port
the chemotherapy
the radiation
the anti-estrogens
the weekly blood draws
After the dry mouth
the dry, grayish skin
the stomach issues
the nausea
the constipation
the fatigue
the memory loss
the hair loss
the brain fog

Cancer took my health and my belief that I would always be whole. Cancer stripped me of everything I thought I was. I was left with a new beginning, a fresh canvas and I got to decide what was going to be a part of my life.

I have often said cancer saved my life. Being torn apart by cancer gave me a new look at myself as I picked up the pieces. Often we hold on to things that no longer work for us. We store things to be saved for use at a later time. That time doesn't always exist after cancer.

I was still a nice person after my cancer diagnosis. I was still a caring, giving person. I looked almost the same. When I looked closely at myself though, I saw someone different. I was no longer willing to accept many of the parts of my life. I was no longer going to just let life happen around me. I was going to live every part of my life. I often hear that same thought from other cancer survivors. They had life changes after cancer.

I was in an unhappy marriage. I left.
I was separated from my parents and siblings. I moved.
I wanted to go back to school. I went.
I wanted to show my children a happy mom. I did.
I wanted to write. I wrote.

The hardest part of taking charge of my life was believing that I could.

Route 5 ... a poem

She woke up
got dressed
walked out the door and no one noticed.
Well, that's not really true.
Maybe I should have said:
She woke up
went to the bathroom
fixed a cup of coffee
washed her face
made up her bed
put on makeup
made another cup of coffee
tried on clothes till she found something that fit
fixed a school lunch for her son
prayed with her sister on the phone
checked email
checked Facebook
tried to write
let the dog out
made another cup of coffee
stopped
went to the window
e x h a l e d
all the stresses and worries
she didn't want them back
so, she didn't inhale
for

a
long time
she had to >inhale< eventually
when she did inhale
she inhaled questions.
Why?
Why isn't anything easy?
Why can't she just leave,
for a short time
not forever
leave.
She has a book on her coffee table called, "The Most Scenic Drives in
America".
She picked up the book
opened it to anywhere...
Washington State
Olympia, WA
Route 5
she gets in her car
she drives
to Walmart.

The Swan

Lone swan on the lake
I can hear her call
But I can't see her
She seems distraught
She keeps calling
into the thick veil
of the morning fog

I woke up this morning, started the coffee, turned on the computer and opened the curtains in the living room. As I looked out at the lake, I was mesmerized by the thick fog covering the lake. I quickly poured a cup of coffee and went outside to sit. The air was crisp and fresh. The air felt thick. I felt it entering my body as I inhaled. It woke up all the parts of me that were still groggy. My mind cleared, my eyes took in everything around me and I could breath. I could feel my lungs reaching full capacity with each inhalation.

It felt great to be alive. The sounds of the morning surrounded me: crickets, frogs, birds and a lone swan. I sat on my front porch watching and listening to nothing in particular. The fog on the lake this morning was the thickest I had seen. I couldn't see the water at all. As I sat mesmerized, the swan came near the edge of the lake – right in front of where I was sitting. She moved, moved back and forth in front of me. She sounded desperate, calling out into early morning hours. She continued to disrupt my peaceful morning sounds with her cries but at the same time, she seemed to connect with me.

I had to remain here with her. How long did I sit there? I don't know.

The day was beginning. The fog was lifting. She made one last pass in front of me, and then moved off into center of the lake. As the fog dissipated, I began to see the water. It was flawless and still.

There were reflections of the surrounding houses and trees in the lake. As the swan cut across the lake, everything became clear. She swam with ease and grace. She calmed. She was at peace. I inhaled the desperation I had felt earlier then forcefully exhaled. I calmed and was at peace too.

Carefree ... a poem

I was going through treatments for breast cancer in 2006-2007. I worked so hard to be the same person I was B.C. – before cancer. I remember how challenging it was to be happy all the time. Strong, I could do, but maintaining my perky attitude was hard.

Alone
in a house full of people.
Alone
in a crowd.
Alone
in my mind and my thoughts.

They laugh.
They joke.
They play.
They are carefree.

I want that.
I am supposed to be that,
that is how I have been raised,
raised to know how to behave in life.
I need to be around people.
I need to be talking constantly.

Don't I?
Shouldn't I?

Is something wrong with me if I don't want to smile and perform?
Can I just be alone with my cancer, for a minute?
Can I just be mad and scared?

"What's wrong with you?" they ask.
"Who made you mad?" they prod.

Nothing.
No one.
I just need to be alone.
I need to be alone to find that perfect disposition they seek
     to find that person I am supposed to be.

If I can be alone
I will slap the required smile onto my face.

I will laugh.
I will joke.
I will play.
I will be carefree.
But I will still be alone
they just won't see.

Granny's Cedar Chest

Granny's cedar chest was full of beautiful things she had collected over the years. Things that were "too special" to use. She was saving them for the perfect occasion. Granny had an eye for a bargain, but more than that, she had an eye for things that were unique and beautiful. She found many of her treasures in stores, though many were family items. When she brought something new home she took great care to place it in the cedar chest where it would remain safe, in perfect condition and ready for use on that perfect, special occasion.

When my Granny died, I went through her cedar chests with my father – she had several by then. It made me cry to see the glorious treasure she had carefully and lovingly collected over the years. Treasure she never enjoyed. I suppose she enjoyed knowing she possessed it, but she never took it out and used it. I have wondered about this over the years.

Was this treasure of hers special to her just because she had it? Did she ever own anything she wanted to use? Did she look at some of her treasure and have a memory that went along with it? Why was it so important to have beautiful things that sit in her vault unused?

I believe that Granny enjoyed the search for treasure. I believe she enjoyed knowing it was there. Though the thought of unused treasure – waiting for a special occasion – makes me sad, maybe just knowing it was there was all the pleasure she wanted from her treasure.

I look inside myself often, searching for answers to questions about myself. Why does it bother me so much that Granny never used any of these beautiful things? I think about parts of myself I have hidden away like a treasure "too perfect" to get out of my treasure chest.

I have spent years collecting my dreams and carefully placing them in my treasure chest. Here in my treasure chest, my dreams will remain safe. They will remain in perfect condition never to be found fault with; never to be shattered into a million delicate pieces. Here my dreams remain a possibility.

Do I dare take them out? Maybe if I just take out one of them and try it on for size. Could I do that? Could I trust myself to be careful with one of my dreams? If the dream gets tattered or tarnished, I can still keep it. It will still be beautiful in my eyes. Maybe a bit of wear and tear will change it into something more beautiful than I could have imagined. Maybe just taking it out and letting it have the opportunity for fulfillment will turn it into something incredible;

Something beyond my wildest dreams.

Yoga for Hope

I hope.
I always hope.
Hope for health.
Hope for joy.
Hope for happiness.
Hope helps when we are challenged.
Hope is still there even when we feel all hope is gone.
Hope.

Poses:

Child's pose
½ Camel pose
Plank
Downward Facing Dog
Warrior 1
Warrior 2
Warrior 3
Half Moon Pose

Childs pose is a wonderful place to start. Take your knees out wide and let your body fall gently towards the mat, rest your forehead on the back of your hands. Breathe. Slide your left arm back to your left heel as you move into a ½ Camel Pose on each side. Move to Plank pose then Downward Facing Dog. Step your left foot forward to Warrior 1 and lift your chest towards the sky, add Warrior 2, and Warrior 3. Move to Half Moon Pose if you are feeling balanced, move back to

Downward Facing Dog and repeat on the other side. Make your way back to Downward Facing Dog and then Childs pose. Repeat as often as you would like. I love heart opening poses for hope. This is a flow to allow you to surrender and let hope have a place in your heart.

Yoga Practice Notes

Yoga for Hope

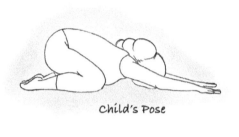

Child's Pose

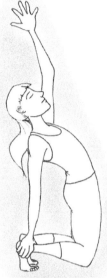

Half Camel Pose

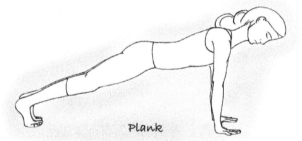

Plank

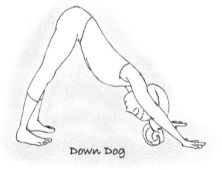

Down Dog

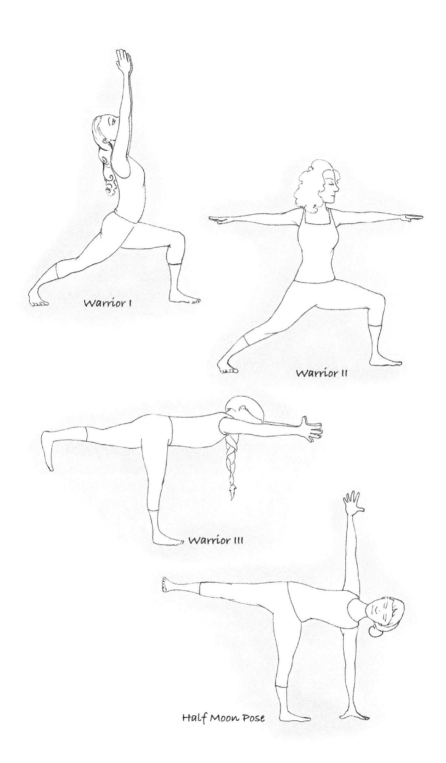

Warrior I

Warrior II

Warrior III

Half Moon Pose

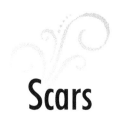

Scars

I have scars. The scars on my body don't bother me. I once thought they would. I once worried that I would be ugly with some of my scars. My surface scars represent someone who has experienced life, the good and the bad.

I have a scar on my knee from falling off my pony, Buttermilk. When I see this scar, I think of her. On my other knee, I have a scar from college when I worked at UPS loading packages. We all have scars on our knees.

There is a scar on my left wrist from tendinitis surgery. When my ex-husband was gone to Egypt for 6 months, I thought it would be a brilliant idea to do 150 full pushups each night. Guess what? Not such a good idea. This scar helps me to remember my body has its limits and if I push those limits my body just might say no.

I have a small scar under my thumb. I sliced my thumb cutting peaches – this scar reminds me to pay attention to details.

I have three scars from breast cancer. There is one on the upper right side of my chest, where the surgeon inserted the venous port - the place where the chemotherapy would enter my body. I have another scar on the inside, cleavage area, of my left breast. This is where the surgeon took out the cancer that threatened me. Under my left arm, I have a scar where they biopsied a lymph node to make sure my cancer hadn't spread to other parts of my body. All of my cancer scars are ugly, but I don't mind them. They are a reminder to me that I can face something terrible and be ok. They remind me of how strong I am. They remind me of the loving prayers that came my way from so many people. They remind me that I am alive.

The scars I have that no one sees are the scars that cause me the most pain. These are the mental scars that represent loss of trust, disillusionment, a callused heart and despair. Those scars are there because I was treated like I had no value, because I allowed myself to be treated poorly. Some of those scars I caused all by myself. My poor judgment left me with scars that threatened to never heal.

Scars I bear because of choices I made or did not make – those are the scars I felt every day. Those were the scars that threatened to tear me apart. Those scars made me question myself. I didn't want any more scars like those so I micro-managed my emotions. I worked hard to keep myself from being hurt. Those scars are healed now but the memory of them remain in the back of my mind.

I hoped one day to be free of that fear. I hoped one day to be able to trust fully. I hoped one day to be able to love with my whole heart. I knew that day would be the day the scars on the inside of me would be healed. I have grown into who I am from those scars.

Yellow Pajamas ... a poem

I watch you
    as you ignore me.
I listen to you breathe
    as you find everything more interesting than me.
I bought new pajamas
    you didn't notice.
They are yellow flannel with little blue flowers.
Happy.
Cozy.
Ignored.
Just like me.

Do You Exist? ... a poem

I woke up this morning and felt you thinking about me.
I felt your arms around me. I felt you kiss my neck.

I woke up this morning and felt you with me.
Did you wake me up? Or did I wake you?

Who are you?
You are not here but I can feel you near me.

Were you made for me, like I was made for you?
Do you exist, or have I just imagined you?

Have I just wanted you to "be" so much that I created you in my mind?
Are you a fairy tale?

I have searched for you all my life.
I have needed you even when I didn't know I needed you.

I needed you when I was searching for who I was after my parents divorced.
You could have been the one I leaned on as my world was destroyed.

I needed you when I was surrounded by people but still felt alone.
You could have been the person that made me feel accepted.

I needed you when I had breast cancer.
You could have been my support. You could have given me hope.

You could have given me love, and you could have told me I would be ok.
You could have dried my tears. You could have been my strength.

I have wanted you for a long time.
I want you to hear what I have to say.

I want you to warm me when I am cold.
I want you to be mine.

Are you searching for me too?
Are you loving me and don't know it yet?

Did you wake me this morning
or did I wake you?

Peace

It's quiet in the yoga studio this morning. The only sounds are my inhales and exhales. Sitting on my mat. Soft glow of the lights in the corners of the room. Inhale. Exhale. Peace. Calm. Contentment.

I love owning a yoga studio with my sister, Lauren. We hoped for years to be able to work in a business together. We wanted to create something that felt real to us, something that included our love of helping others and helping people to find joy in their lives. We did it. This place is perfect, and we love our yogis.

I'm waiting for the first of my yoga students to arrive. They don't come in quietly. I never encourage that. I want to feel the life in each person as they arrive. They may or may not say a word, but their energies are full. They are present.

When I first began teaching yoga, I noticed that many of my students came to yoga because they were healing something: a hurt shoulder, a knee, a back, a wrist. Or they came because they could no longer do their favorite activity and were looking for something to fill that void. Some people found yoga through their doctors, their friends or maybe they saw an article in a magazine about the benefits of yoga and wanted to give it a try.

However, they got here doesn't matter.
They came for
        fitness
        stress release

weight loss
support
friendship
community
flexibility

They came, and we are here to support them. Yogi's are different. They want to be in shape, they want to change their world and they want to be a part of something more than themselves. Yoga will help get them in shape physically and mentally. Our yogi's change their piece of the world; they make a difference in the lives of the people around them. They come to yoga for all kinds of reasons and they grow and improve.

I sit, and I wait. I love this time before they arrive to take a few breaths and remember how grateful I am for this life I have. I love, and I am loved. I hear the car doors closing. I hear the joy in the voices outside of the studio. I love the life my students bring into the studio. We tell them this is our studio. Lauren and I built it and filled it with our love and joy. They bring their own love and joy. Together we have created something special.

Peace
Calm
Contentment
Gratitude
Joy

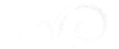

Her Face

I can see her face - the real person, alive and moving.
I got back from a convention in San Diego Saturday night. I was gone for a week. I didn't check the sign-in's last week for the yoga classes while I was gone. If I had, I would have noticed that one particular yogi had not been in class all week. We don't monitor all the students and their attendance but there are a few people that always let us know when they are going to miss class. She is one of those yogis.

Her daughter, Paula, is about my age. She has a beautiful face and her spirit is even more beautiful. Paula's husband was in the Air Force for a while and they were stationed at Reese Air Force Base in Lubbock, Texas. My ex-husband was the head of the Military Science department at Texas Technological University in Lubbock, Texas. We didn't live in Lubbock at the same time but we both knew what it was like to live in a place where the people are wonderful, and the landscape is flat and brown with dust storms sprinkled in for good measure. Paula and I both have two children. We love a nice lunch out. We laugh. We care. We both fought breast cancer.

My sister, Lauren called me Sunday morning to let me know that Paula's cancer had progressed and had metastasized to her brain. She didn't want to tell me when I was out of town. She seemed to know how it would affect me. Do you know that feeling when you momentarily freeze, when your heart hurts and you just have to let it hurt? I slowly sank down to the floor and cried. Lauren let me cry. I cried for our yogi, for Paula and for Paula's daughter whom I also had in my yoga classes. I cried because of the fear I knew they were feeling. I cried out of fear I was feeling for myself and for other women that come to the studio that have had breast cancer. I cried in sadness and I cried in anger.

I kept Paula in my thoughts all day Sunday. I drove to the studio the next morning to teach a class. Linda was the first yogi to arrive. She is soft spoken. She does organic gardening. She adores her husband. Linda has had breast cancer twice and also Parkinson's disease. She walked in, sat her bag down, hugged me and cried. She cried for our yogi and Paula, and she cried in fear for herself and for me. She told me how mad she is right now at cancer, at Parkinson's and at having to worry about her health all the time.

I thought it was just me. Just me that was numb and scared and pissed off. I see other breast cancer patients and survivors moving through their life, but I don't know what they are feeling inside. I don't ask. Are they like me? Are they like Linda? Are they mad at cancer too? Are they grateful to have their lives? Did cancer give them a reason to look at how they were living their life and make positive changes like I did? Talking to Linda and seeing that she had the same fear and anger at cancer hovering right on the surface of her emotions that morning was eye-opening for me. It made me wonder if all the sweet, pink-ribboned survivors are walking around with a smile on their lips and a touch of fear and anger in their hearts.

Linda and I hugged and felt the heavy fear and desperation. We worried about Paula and ourselves. We felt guilt for worrying about ourselves when Paula was fighting for her life. It could have easily been us. We were lucky, our cancer was gone. We hope and pray that it won't come back, but we're always scared that it might.

The Knitted Cap

We were so exhausted from the fun of Disney World; the airline flight, eating out, laughing, walking, tons of walking...the magic of Disney. This was our first Mother/Daughter trip in 8 years - our first trip since...the knitted cap.

It felt good to be back in Tennessee. Samantha, laughed as I wandered around the parking garage at the airport pushing the key fob, hoping my car would tell me where it was. Found the car. It was still there. We loaded the car with our luggage. Samantha had put together a playlist for our trip, songs we loved to sing. As I backed the car out, she punched in NSYNC. We couldn't stop laughing as she sang every word to Space Cowboy perfectly. Coming up for air, we realized we were famished. We stopped at Einstein's Bagels. We walked up to the counter and ordered coffee and a bagel. Laughter. Music. Mother/Daughter time. Memories.

Then I noticed Her. I noticed the beautiful woman sitting beside us. She was thirty-something, had two gorgeous daughters with her (about five & seven) and her husband. She was the mother in a perfect family portrait. I couldn't give you many details about her looks. I didn't notice the color of her eyes. Though I did notice the smile on her lips did not quite reach her eyes. She had porcelain skin and a slim build. But I don't' remember the shape of her face. I noticed her because of the knitted cap that covered her head - her bald head. I wasn't hungry anymore. I wanted to go hug her and tell her she would be ok, because I was ok. I wanted to tell her I understood how scared she was. I needed her to know that.

I felt empty watching her. The memories of what I had gone through came rushing back. I had a hole in my stomach, a void, a fear. Fear for myself and for her. I felt as though I had failed her and all others going through cancer. I failed them because I had not shared my story.

I glanced up at Samantha. She had a tear in her eye.

So, Did I live Happily Ever After?

I ask this because when I was going through my treatments and searching for books that would tell me how various stages felt – most of them ended with a happily ever after. I love happy endings when I'm at a movie or reading a novel. Real life doesn't always have happy endings.

When I was walking down the hallway to check on my children after telling them I had cancer, I wasn't thinking about happy anything. When I was going to my first chemo treatment, I was just plain scared. There was not a lot of happy mixed in. There was some "let's get this over with" mixed in with fear, but happy was on holiday break. On day 20 of radiation, fear was still the headliner but shared top billing with anxiety.

Even today, when I know my mammogram appointment is getting near, happy wants to be silent. The difference between today and when I was going through treatment is noticeable. I'm a different person. I've changed. I'm also not going through the treatments anymore.

I wonder if people will look back 100 years from now and be horrified at the poison and radiation of cancer treatments, taking a patient's body as close to destruction as possible, then waiting for any positive results. I had great doctors and wonderful, caring nurses and staff taking care of me as I battled cancer. I hope easier treatments are in the future for the next generations though.

I had breakfast recently with one of my friends who also happens to be one of my yoga instructors. Linda is a two-time breast cancer survivor.

Linda is a beautiful soul. We sat at Kali's Diner, Linda with a pancake and an egg and me with a ½ order of French toast, both of us with lots of coffee. We talked about yoga, my recent trips, her upcoming guests, the horrible insurance system. Then she asked me if I ever thought about why some people get cancer and survive and some don't. I knew she was talking about one of the yogi's who recently died after a long battle with cancer. We looked at each other. We didn't have to say anything else. The fear was there. It will always be there, but we can't let it be the focus of our lives. We had an in-depth conversation silently. We did everything right and we still got breast cancer. We are both still here.

But did I live happily ever after?

I am healthy. I am now married to a man I am completely in love with, who loves me completely. My children are healthy and happy. I own a yoga studio with my sister and we are connecting with beautiful souls through yoga. I help other people believe in themselves. I am a writer. I believe in myself.

I am happy.

Yoga Flows

Yoga for Anger

Anger and fear took turns being in charge during this time. I was scared then I was angry. I was scared that I would not be okay. I was angry that I had done everything right and I still got cancer. I ate right, and I exercised. Wasn't that supposed to keep me healthy? My rational side knew that cancer was random, but my irrational side was mad.

It is hard to hold anger and kindness in the same hand.
Affirmation: I am kind.

Sun Salutation A

- Mountain
- Forward Fold
- Monkey
- Plank
- Updog
- Down dog
- Forward fold
- Mountain

When you have exhausted your anger:
Seated Forward Fold, Easy Seat with a focus on your breath and finish with Legs Up the Wall Pose.

Sun salutation A can be a complete practice alone. It can stretch, strengthen and relax the body. This practice can also reduce anger and stress. Sun salutations are generally used to energize the body, but they can also be done in such a way that relaxes the body.

To do Sun Salute A: Begin in Mountain pose, breathe. Reach your arms up towards the sky, noticing how your body feels, Forward Fold. Release the back of the body and release the anger and fear. Flatten your back and hold your belly in as you move to Monkey pose. Step back into plank or modified plank, lower your body down to Upward Facing Dog or modified Cobra. Move to Downward Facing Dog, let your back body stretch. Remember, Downward Facing Dog is a resting pose, when you are ready, step back in to a Forward Fold then lift back up into Mountain Pose. Continue this flow until you are ready to move into Legs Up the Wall Pose.

Yoga Practice Notes

_____

_____

_____

_____

_____

_____

_____

_____

_____

_____

_____

_____

_____

_____

_____

_____

_____

_____

_____

Yoga for Anger

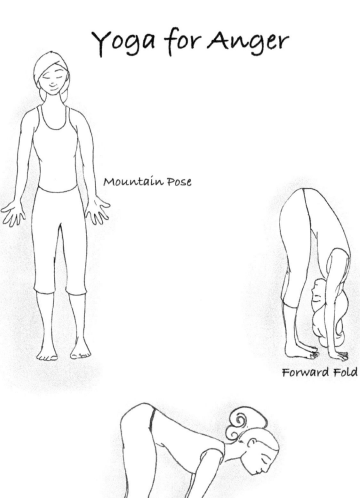

Mountain Pose

Forward Fold

Monkey Pose

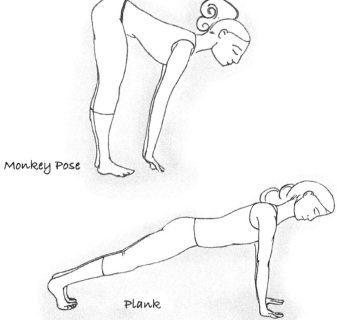

Plank

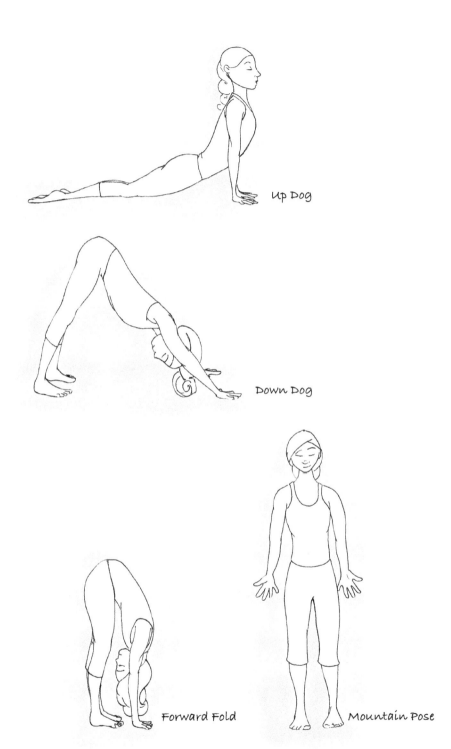

Up Dog

Down Dog

Forward Fold

Mountain Pose

Yoga for Chemo Brain

Chemo brain, for me, was real and it was scary. I felt like I was living in a fog. I could not remember things. I had trouble focusing on what I was reading. My mind would wander, and I would have to re-read. Yoga may help with chemo brain, with your balance and with your memory.

For this flow use the Hakini mudra when you are in the poses. To do this mudra, bring your hands in front of your body, palms facing. Bring your fingertips of both hands together and allow them to lightly touch. This mudra helps with memory and concentration.

Affirmation: I am focused

Poses:

Mountain pose
Eagle, both sides
Chair pose
Crescent Lunge pose
Tree pose

Mountain pose makes you feel grounded. Eagle is a balancing and focusing pose. Chair pose helps you to feel strong. Crescent Lunge pose helps you to feel flexible and allows you to work on your balance. Tree pose is a balancing pose and a grounding pose. The intention of this pose it to feel strong, balanced and grounded.

Start in Mountain, breathe until you are ready to move. Slowly sit into Chair pose. Find your focus and balance before you move into Crescent Lunge pose. From Crescent Lunge, slowly move into Tree pose allowing your breath to move with your body. Breathe and balance, then move back to Mountain pose. Repeat other side
Flow through this short flow until you feel focused.

Move into meditation.

Yoga for Chemo Brain

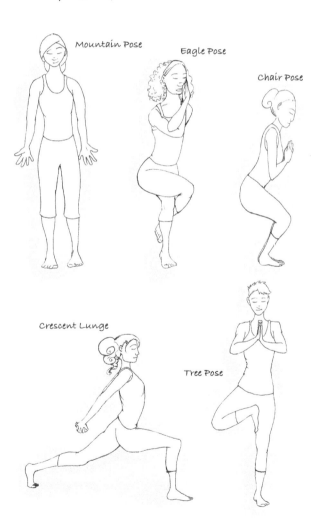

Mountain Pose

Eagle Pose

Chair Pose

Crescent Lunge

Tree Pose

Yoga for Constipation

The treatments for cancer have many side effects. Some chemotherapy drugs and radiation can cause constipation. I dealt with this during chemo and radiation. These yoga poses helped me. Move into each pose and stay there as long as it feels good to you. If you need a time, stay with each pose for 8 inhalations or more.

Affirmation: I am balanced

Poses:

Easy Seat Pose with deep breathing and/or meditation. You may want to add a twist to each side if that is comfortable.

Forward Fold, Ragdoll Arms.

Downward Facing Dog

Lying spinal twist

Seated deep breathing and/or mediation helped to calm the stress and helped improve elimination. Forward fold calms the body and compresses the abdominal area. This can help with digestion. Downward facing dog is a full body stretch and helps to release tension. Lying spinal twist helps with bloating and gas. This pose is a great combination of a twist and a resting pose. Do each of these poses as a stand-alone. Stay with them as long as it feels good to you.

Constipation can happen anytime. I have found that I get constipated when I am stressed. Some chemotherapy drugs and some pain medication can have constipation as a side effect.

Yoga for Constipation

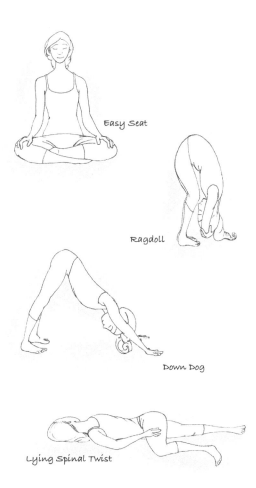

Easy Seat

Ragdoll

Down Dog

Lying Spinal Twist

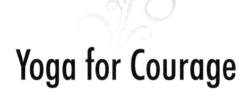

Yoga for Courage

You need courage to get through diagnosis, treatment and recovery from breast cancer treatments. I love the chest opening and back bending aspects of sun salute C. Moving from child's pose to ½ camel you feel the release of child's pose and the heart opening of camel. Try this flow when you need a shot of courage.

Affirmation: I am courageous

Poses:

Sun Salute C,
Mountain pose, reach up standing backbend
Forward fold
Crescent Lunge, right leg in front
Plank
Upward Facing Dog
Downward Facing Dog
Crescent Lunge, left leg in front
Forward Fold
Standing Backbend back to Mountain Pose

Sun Salute C, repeat 2 times with a low lunge
Sun Salute C, repeat 4 times with a crescent lunge
Mountain Pose – say to yourself I am, on the inhale and courageous, on the exhale.

Move to child's pose with arms extended out in front

Slide left arm back to left heel as you come up to ½ camel pose
Move back to extended child's pose
Slide right arm back to right heel as you come up to ½ camel pose
Repeat this flow slowly, 2-8 times on each side

Move to a wide legged child's pose with your forehead on your two fists and breath.
Breath in, I am and exhale, courageous.

Yoga for Courage
Sun Salute C

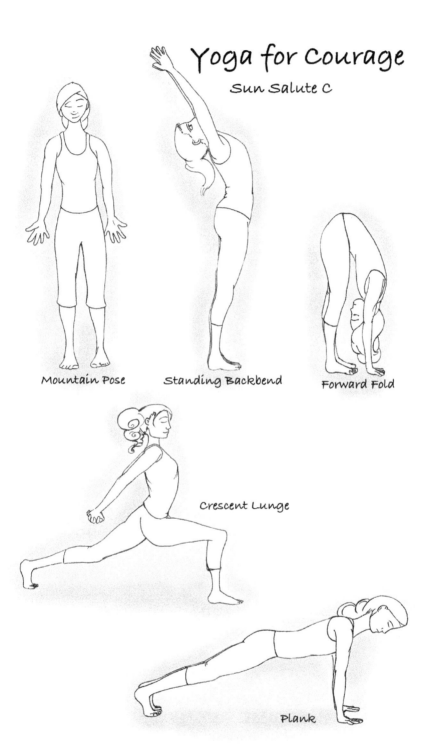

Mountain Pose   Standing Backbend   Forward Fold

Crescent Lunge

Plank

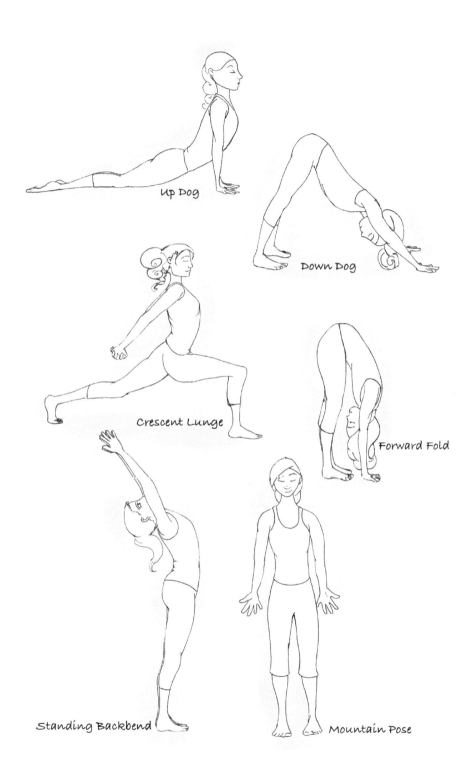

Up Dog

Down Dog

Crescent Lunge

Forward Fold

Standing Backbend

Mountain Pose

Yoga for Courage Continued

Heart Opening Flow

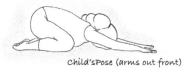

Child'sPose (arms out front)

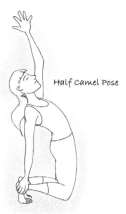

Half Camel Pose

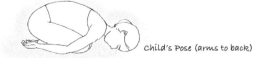

Child's Pose (arms to back)

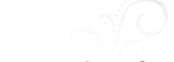

Yoga Flow for Fear

Yoga will relieve your fear. Really? It will not but it will help you better cope with fear.

Try alternate nostril breathing before you begin this flow.

Beginning in an easy seated position, focus on your breath. As you breathe in, say to yourself, *I am ...* as you exhale, say to yourself, *calm.* Continue breathing like this for as long as you would like. Slowly move onto your hands and knees for Cat/Cow pose. Continue moving through the poses while focusing on your inhalations and exhalations. Breathing in, *I am* and exhaling, *calm.*

Affirmation– I am Calm

Poses:
Cat/Cow -
Downward Facing Dog
Plank – modified and/or full
Side plank
Forward Fold with rag doll arms (modification, knees bent)

Cat/Cow helps to get your body moving. I love the feeling of waking up the torso. In Cow pose I breathe in strength and in cat I exhale fear. Downward Facing Dog and Plank remind me that I am strong. Side Plank keeps me balanced and Forward Fold allows me to release the fears. These poses can be done individually, or you can repeat them in a flow. In a flow, you can rest in Downward Facing Dog between each pose.

Yoga For Fear

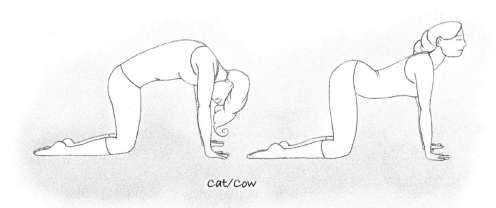

Cat/Cow

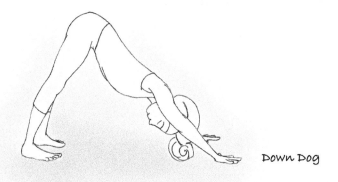

Down Dog

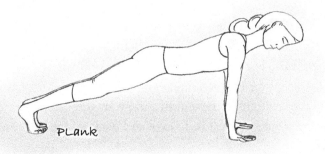

Plank

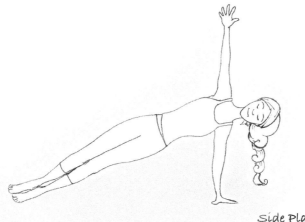

Side Plank

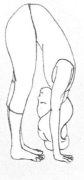

Forward Fold

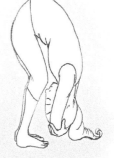

Ragdoll

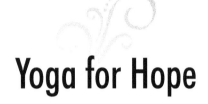

Yoga for Hope

I hope.
I always hope.
Hope for health.
Hope for joy.
Hope for happiness.
Hope helps when we are challenged.
Hope is still there even when we feel all hope is gone.
Hope.

Poses:

Child's pose
½ Camel pose
Plank
Downward Facing Dog
Warrior 1
Warrior 2
Warrior 3
Half Moon Pose

Childs pose is a wonderful place to start. Take your knees out wide and let your body fall gently towards the mat, rest your forehead on the back of your hands. Breathe. Slide your left arm back to your left heel as you move into a ½ Camel Pose on each side. Move to Plank pose then Downward Facing Dog. Step your left foot forward to Warrior 1 and lift your chest towards the sky, add Warrior 2, and Warrior 3. Move to Half Moon Pose if you are feeling balanced, move back to

Downward Facing Dog and repeat on the other side. Make your way back to Downward Facing Dog and then Childs pose. Repeat as often as you would like. I love heart opening poses for hope. This is a flow to allow you to surrender and let hope have a place in your heart.

Yoga for Hope

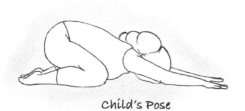

Child's Pose

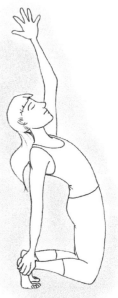

Half Camel Pose

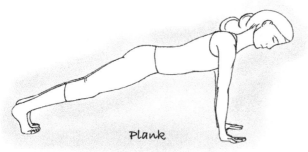

Plank

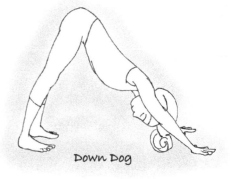

Down Dog

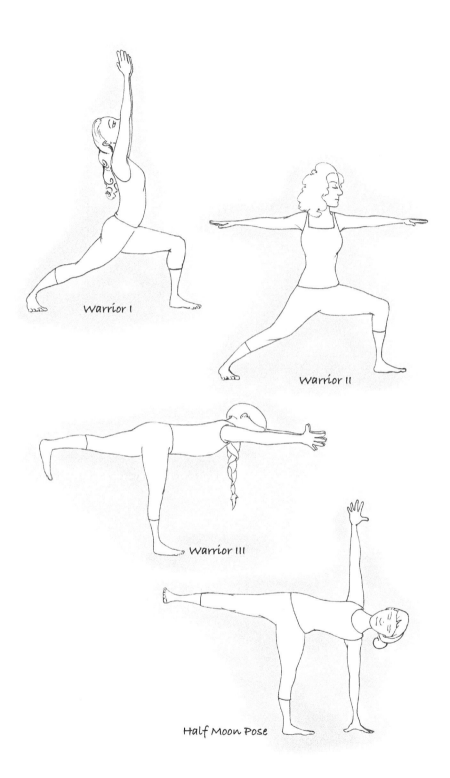

Warrior I

Warrior II

Warrior III

Half Moon Pose

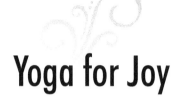

Yoga for Joy

I want to consider myself a joyful person. I am most of the time. I often felt sorry for myself when I was going through breast cancer. Try this flow when you are feeling sad. Repeat each piece of the flow as long as it feels good to you. This flow can give you a release, a feeling of freedom and joy.

Affirmation: I am joyful

Poses:

Mountain Pose
Stretch up to the sky
Grab your right wrist with your left hand and stretch your body to the left
Grab your left wrist with your right hand and stretch your body to the right
Standing backbend – listen to your body.
Repeat

Forward fold
Downward facing dog
Upward facing dog
Forward fold
Repeat 8 times

Flowing ½ camel (extended Childs pose, slide left hand back to left heel, ½ camel – other side)

Repeat 4-8 times, taking your time and breath. Noticing how your feel. Feel your body. You are alive.

Move to downward facing dog
Lunge forward to crescent lunge and clasp hand behind your back (keep elbows bent or straighten) Open to Sun God. Back to crescent lunge. Downward facing dog.
Repeat other side.

Reclined bound angle
Knees to chest
Lying spinal twist each side

When you have finished the flow, lie down on your mat for relaxation. Savasana is not nap time though I do have students that have fallen asleep. The intent is to stay alert but relaxed. This is hard for many students but is helpful to everyone, especially for cancer patients. I like to have my students open their palms to the ceiling and let their legs flop out. As you lie in relaxation pose allow your muscles to release. This is a time for you, don't cheat yourself out of this part of your practice.

Yoga For Joy

Flow A

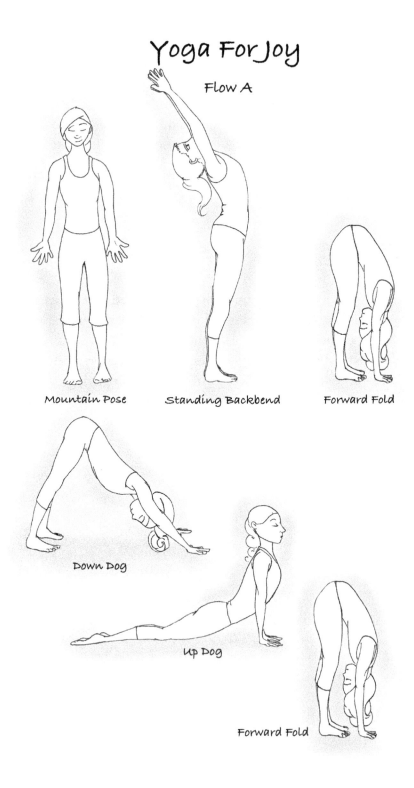

Mountain Pose

Standing Backbend

Forward Fold

Down Dog

Up Dog

Forward Fold

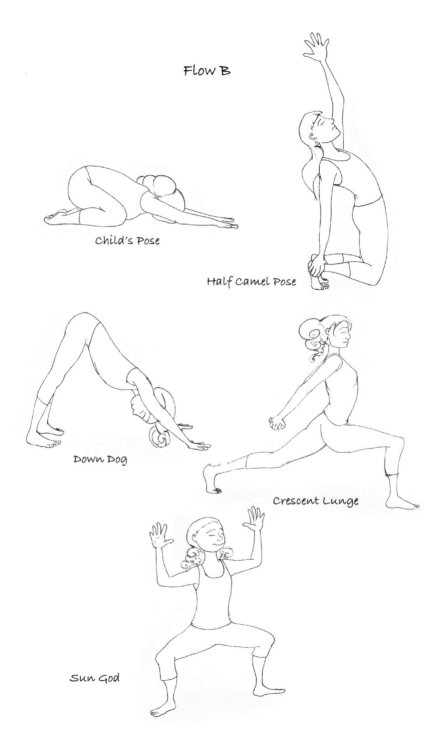

Flow B

Child's Pose

Half Camel Pose

Down Dog

Crescent Lunge

Sun God

Yoga for Joy Continued

Flow C

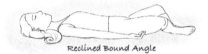
Reclined Bound Angle

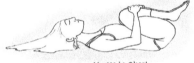
Knees to Chest

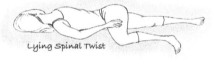
Lying Spinal Twist

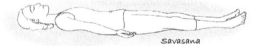
Savasana

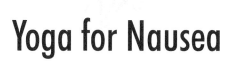

Yoga for Nausea

When you feel nauseous, the last thing you want to do is move around a great deal. The poses in this flow are meant to relax and relieve your body.

Affirmation: I am grounded

Poses:

Easy Seat

Bound angle

Legs up the wall

Easy seat is a hip opener and helps to reduce stress and anxiety.

Bound angle stretches the inner thighs, groins and knees. This is another hip opener, so you can the same stress reduction benefits that you get in easy seat.

When I first started learning to teach yoga. I head from numerous instructors say that the hips were the emotional depot of the body, so releasing your hips helped to relieve a myriad of challenges to include, stress, anxiety and depression. I noticed, in my classes, that it had to a positive effect on my students. If we think about it when we feel stress, a normal reaction might be to curl ourselves into the fetal position. This movement is initiated in the hips and they tighten. So, stretching and releasing can help you to let go of that tension and stress.

Legs up the wall pose looks like a passive pose but it actually an active pose. Most everyone can do this pose, it doesn't require loads of flexibility and strength. This is one of my favorite poses. These poses help to relax you, improve your circulation, can help reduce swelling and it stretches your hamstrings and back.

Yoga for Nausea

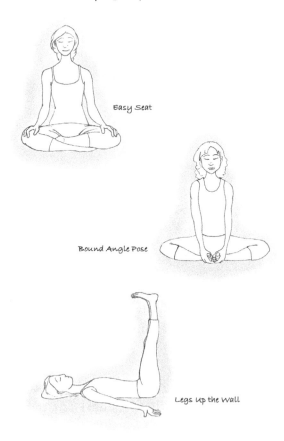

Easy Seat

Bound Angle Pose

Legs Up the Wall

Yoga for Positivity

I didn't always stay positive during treatments for cancer. I am not always positive today. I try to be aware when negativity starts creeping in. I chose the poses in this flow because of the hip opening and energizing benefits of these poses. These poses make me feel better and generally make me less stressed. They help to increase my happiness. Positivity can help to combat negativity.

Affirmation: I am optimistic

Poses:

Sun god to temple, back to sun god then to temple.
Flow to each side 8 times

Add:
Crescent lunge
Warrior I
Tree
Warrior II
Back to Sun God and do the other side

Yoga for Positivity

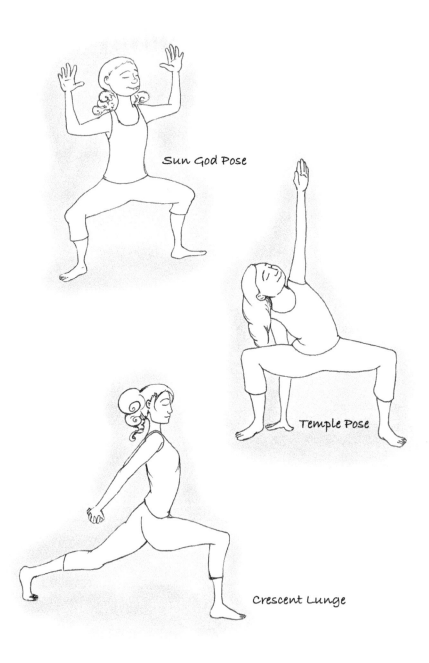

Sun God Pose

Temple Pose

Crescent Lunge

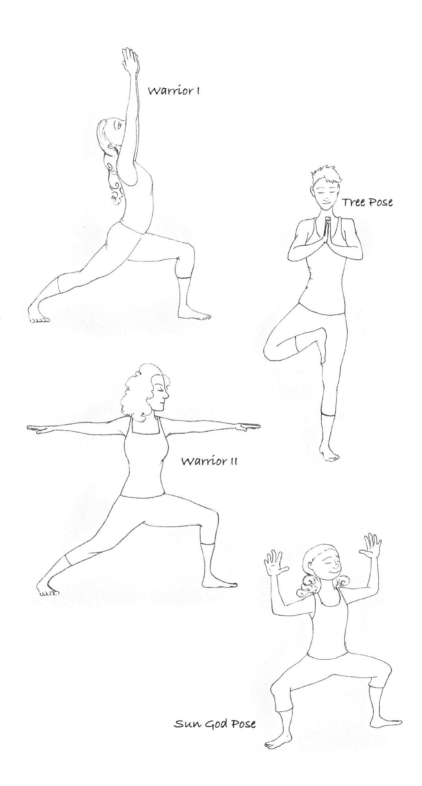

Warrior 1

Tree Pose

Warrior II

Sun God Pose

Self-Acceptance Yoga flow

We all struggle with self-acceptance in some way. Being happy and satisfied with yourself helps you to find more joy in your life.

Affirmation: I am enough
Easy seat – lotus mudra – sit and breath for 8 slow inhalations.

The Lotus Mudra is a grounding mudra. It is a great way to focus on maintaining your foundation and when you have a strong foundation, you have a better chance at self-acceptance. Bring the base of the palms together at the heart center, touching the thumbs and pinky fingers together. Spread the rest of the fingers out like the lotus flower opening toward the sunlight.

Flow:
Child's pose flow – child's pose, come up onto knees (shins on floor), reach arms to the sky, back to child's, repeat 8 times
Downward Dog
Warrior 1, right leg in front, arms out to sides, chest up to sky, inhale
Plank
Updog
Downdog
Back to right leg in front
Open to Sun God
Warrior 1 to other side left leg in front, arms out to sides, chest up to sky, inhale
Plank
Updog

Downdog
Child's pose
Repeat

The way you approach your practice effects the benefits you will reap. I chose these poses because of the way they make you feel mentally and physically.

Childs pose is a place to surrender the self-doubt, even if only for the time you are on your mat. Hopefully, you will remember how free you felt later when you are tempted to pick the self-doubt back up. The poses in this flow help you feel strong, balanced and in control. I love this flow when I want more love and compassion for myself.

Yoga For Self-Acceptance

Warm up to Surrender Self-Doubt

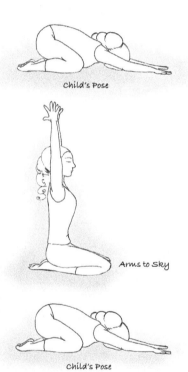

Child's Pose

Arms to Sky

Child's Pose

Yoga Practice Notes

Yoga Flow for Self-Acceptance

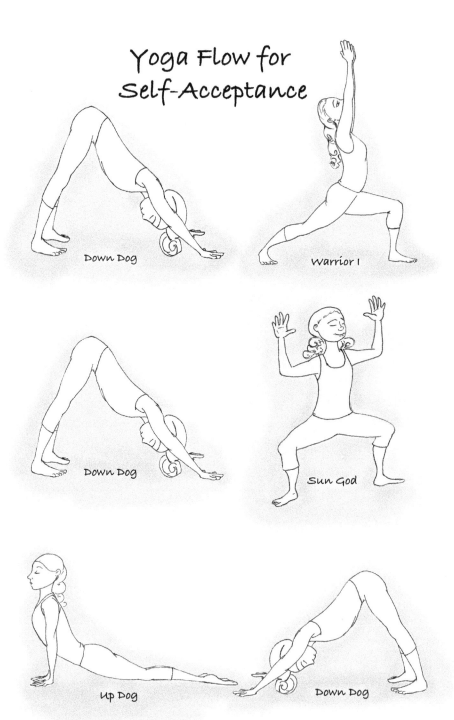

Down Dog

Warrior I

Down Dog

Sun God

Up Dog

Down Dog

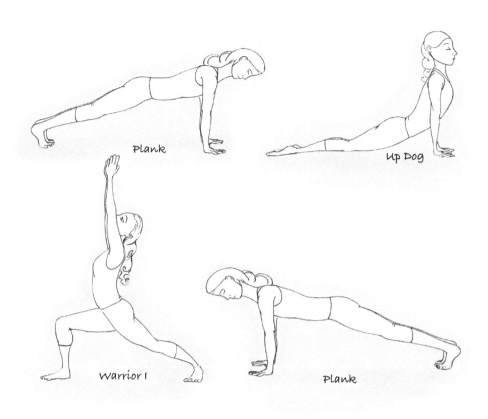

Plank

Up Dog

Warrior I

Plank

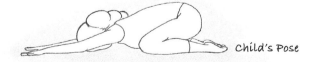

Child's Pose

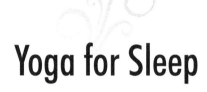

Yoga for Sleep

Many cancer patients experience problems sleeping during and after treatments. I was sleepy for about three days after chemotherapy and exhausted during radiation treatments. I was never a person that took naps, but I would find myself falling asleep if I ever slowed down during the day. The treatments took so much of my strength and disrupted my sleep. I was tired, but I struggled to fall asleep.

Poses:

Easy Seated Forward Fold

Child's pose

Legs up the wall

Lying Spinal Twist

Relax

Easy seated forward bend is an easy pose to get into, opens the hips and relaxes the body. Forward fold can relieve headaches, lower stress and help with insomnia. Child's pose just feels good. There are several ways to do child's pose. You can find the best variation for you. Legs up the wall pose is one of my favorite yoga poses. It helps to improve circulation, relieve headaches and is considered a gentle inversion. This pose helps to relax the body and this makes it easier to relax the mind.

When our body and mind are relaxed we have a better chance of sleeping well. Lying spinal twist relieves tension in the back and helps digestion.

You may also want to try alternate nostril breathing for sleep.

Yoga for Sleep

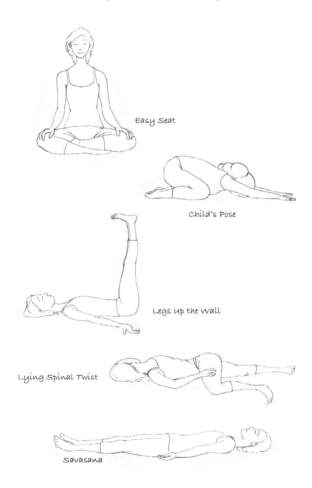

Easy Seat

Child's Pose

Legs Up the Wall

Lying Spinal Twist

Savasana

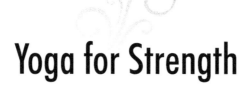

Yoga for Strength

When I began teaching yoga I often heard, "isn't yoga just stretching?". New students were always surprised to find out that yoga could be challenging. It is important to maintain strong bodies. It was especially important to me during cancer treatment. I read that the treatments could cause bone loss, so I wanted to do everything I could to stay strong. This flow is full of strength building poses and should be done at your own pace. The repetitions and times that I have included are suggestions. Remember you should always listen to your own body and work when you need to be each day.

Affirmation: I am strong

Warm-up, Sun Salute A, repeat 3-8 times

Plank – full or modified, 30-60 seconds

Side Plank – full or modified, 10 seconds each side

Downward facing dog, to rest and reset breath

Dolphin, 30 seconds

Forearm plank, 30-60 seconds

Forearms side plank, 10 seconds each side

Childs pose to reset breath

Repeat entire flow, 1 – 5 times

Yoga for Strength
Sun Salute A

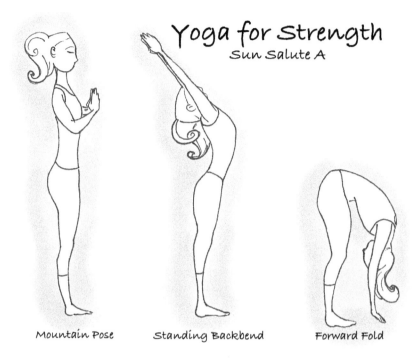

Mountain Pose   Standing Backbend   Forward Fold

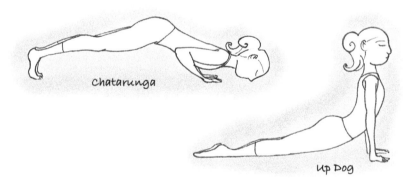

Chatarunga   Up Dog

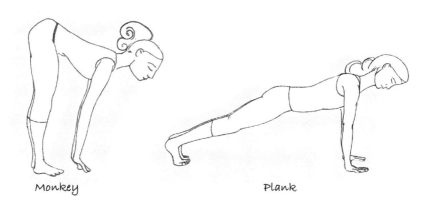

Monkey

Plank

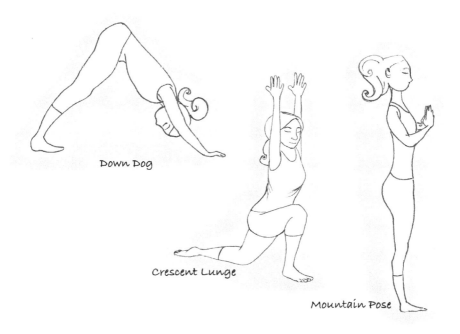

Down Dog

Crescent Lunge

Mountain Pose

Strength Holds

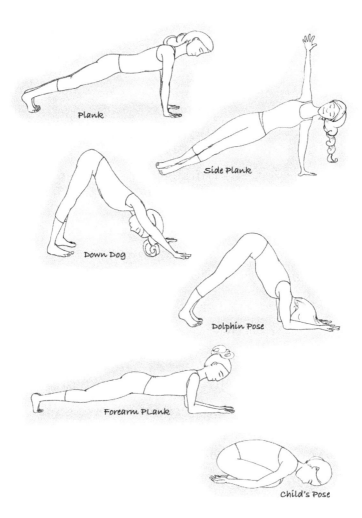

Plank

Side Plank

Down Dog

Dolphin Pose

Forearm Plank

Child's Pose

Yoga for Stress, Anxiety, Depression

Radiation was hard. Radiation took all of my energy. I had been counting on that energy to get me through the treatment. I was left raw and tired. Yoga can help lower your anxiety, depression and stress.

I had a yoga practice in place and it helped tremendously. It did not keep me from feeling tired, stressed, anxiety-laden and raw but it made the side effects easier. I had to be more careful of the poses during this time. I had burns, open sores and aches that I had to work around.

I felt little peace during chemotherapy, but I felt even less during radiation treatment.

Affirmation: I am peace.

Poses:
You can do these individually or put them into a flow together.

Mountain Pose
Reach up to the sky
Chair
Fold down to a Forward Fold
Step back the right foot back to a Low Crescent Lunge – hands on the floor, left leg in front
Plank
Downward Facing Dog

Step forward with the left leg into Warrior II
Crescent lunge
Step into Mountain Pose and do other side.
Flow through these poses as long as it feels good to you.
Move to Seated Forward Fold
Cow Face Pose
Seated Straddle
Reclined Bound Angle
Savasana

Mountain pose was grounding and helped me to feel present. Chair pose, like plank pose and downward facing dog pose reminded me that I am strong. The emotional release of forward fold, the hip opening in Warrior II and the balancing aspect of crescent lunge all helped me stay strong. Seated forward fold stretches the back and hamstrings. Seated straddle pose, and reclined bound angle help to relax and lessen stress.

Doing this flow during radiation will be easier at the beginning of the treatment. As you get further into the treatment, you may find you are uncomfortable with some of the arm movements, modify to make it work for you.

Yoga Practice Notes

_____

_____

_____

_____

_____

_____

_____

_____

_____

_____

_____

_____

_____

_____

_____

_____

_____

_____

Yoga for Stress,

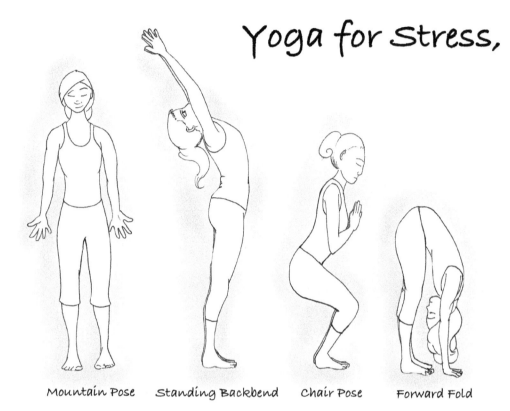

Mountain Pose   Standing Backbend   Chair Pose   Forward Fold

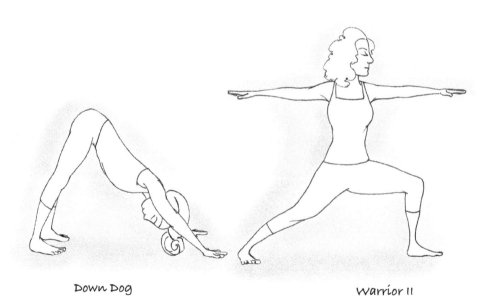

Down Dog   Warrior II

Anxiety, and Depression

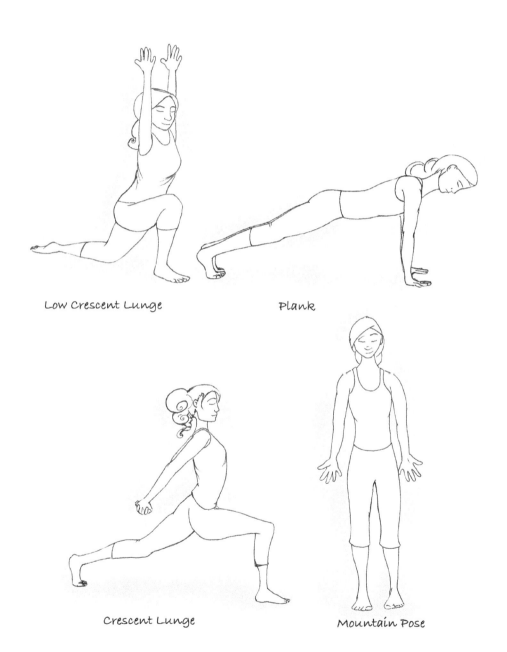

Low Crescent Lunge

Plank

Crescent Lunge

Mountain Pose

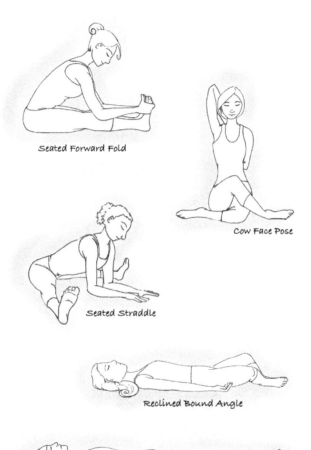

Seated Forward Fold

Cow Face Pose

Seated Straddle

Reclined Bound Angle

Savasana

Yoga after Breast Cancer Surgery

After you have surgery for breast cancer you may have a decrease in the range of motion in your arm and shoulder. This will vary depending on if you have a biopsy, lymph node biopsy, lumpectomy, mastectomy and/or breast reconstruction. You will not want to do any of these exercises without first getting permission from your doctor. Remember, you need to always listen to your body when you exercise. Start slowly. Add poses as they feel comfortable.

Affirmation: I am whole

Poses:

Mountain to Forward fold. Add, standing backbends as you flow. Repeat 8+ times.
Add Eagle on each side when you get ready to change sides
Add Crescent after the eagle on each side.

Take your time. Full inhales and exhales in each pose before you add the next.
As you feel more comfortable, open arms to sides and lift chest in crescent.

Flow through these poses until you feel ready to move to downward facing dog. Notice how you feel in downward facing dog.

Move to the floor. Focused breath for 2 minutes.
Cow Face Pose

Savasana

Mountain pose is a strong grounding pose. You need that after surgery. Stay in this pose for several breaths. Forward fold is a nice releasing pose for me. I love to dive towards the floor and release the worries and tension. Eagle pose helps to feel balanced though you may not be able to add the arms soon after surgery. The concentration required for eagle is great to help take you mind off the surgery. The arms are moving to the midline of the body, so this pose should be accessible.

Downward facing dog helps to remind you that you are strong but remember to listen to your body. Cow face pose will help you start working on your range of motion after surgery, make sure you are take your time moving deeper into this pose.

Yoga Practice Notes

Yoga after Breast Cancer Surgery

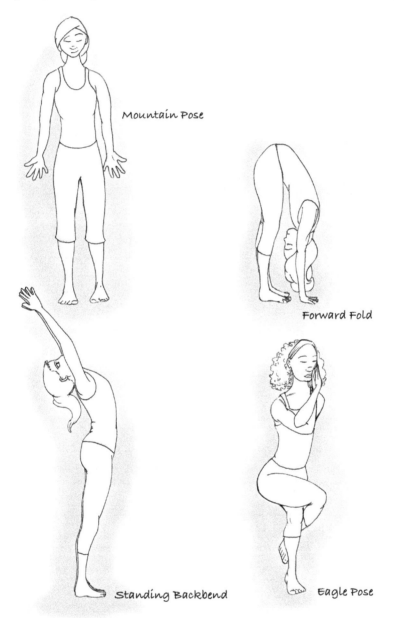

Mountain Pose

Forward Fold

Standing Backbend

Eagle Pose

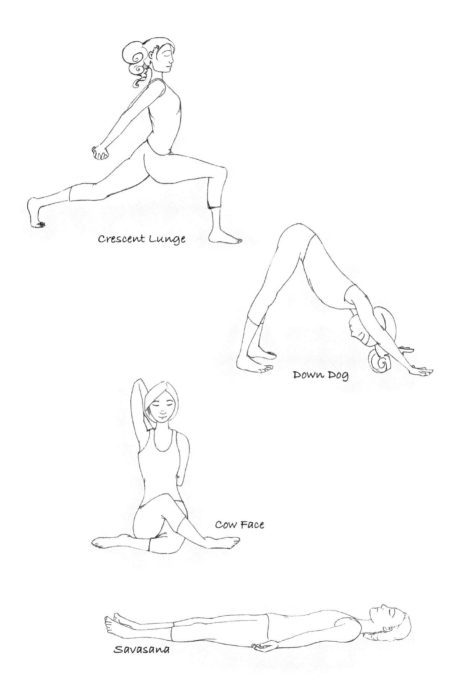

Crescent Lunge

Down Dog

Cow Face

Savasana

Yoga Poses

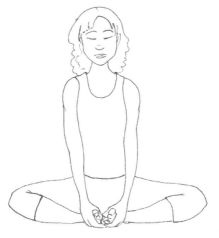

Bound Angle Pose

Bound Angle

A nice release for tight hips and it stretches the inner thighs, groin muscles, and knees.

Begin seated with your legs out in front of you. Bend your knees and gently pull your heels towards your pelvis, drop your knees out to the sides and press the soles of your feet together. Your heels will be about twelve inches from your pelvis.

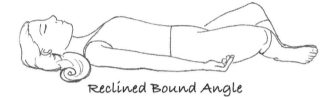

Reclined Bound Angle

Bound Angle, reclined

Stretches tight hips, inner thighs, groin muscles and muscles around the knees.

Begin lying down with your legs out in front of you. Bend your knees and gently pull your heels towards your pelvis, drop your knees out to the sides and press the soles of your feet together. Your heels will be about twelve inches from your pelvis.

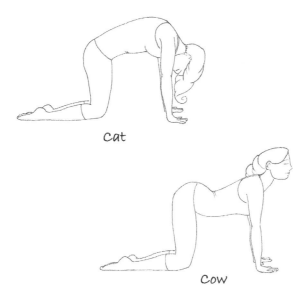

Cat

Cow

Cat/Cow

Warm-up for the torso and stretches the back and neck

Start on your hands and knees in a tabletop position. Your hips are directly above your knees and your wrists, elbows and shoulders are aligned. Your head is in a neutral position. For the "Cat" part of this pose, you will exhale and round your spine towards the ceiling. You will maintain the position of the hips, knees, shoulders and arms as you gently let your head drop. The "Cow" part of this pose, you will inhale and lift your buttocks and chest towards the ceiling while allowing your belly to drop towards the floor. Your head lifts and looks forward or slightly up.

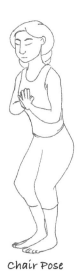
Chair Pose

Chair (arms up or arms at heart center)

Energizes the entire body, Stretches the back of the legs and calves. Strengthens the Achilles tendons, ankles and thigh muscles. A great muscle toning pose for the butt, hips and thighs

Squat down like you are almost sitting in a chair. You have a fist distance between your knees and between your feet. Keep your knees behind your toes and engaging your belly.

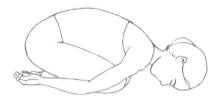

Child's Pose, Arms to Heels

Child's Pose (arms extended out front or at heels)

Rejuvenates the body and engages the back and spine. It helps to refocus your body, mind and breath.

From your hands and knees, point your toes so the tops of your feet are flat on the floor. Shift your body weight back so that your booty rests on your heels. Keep your toes together and knees together or widen your knees so your body can easily drop between your knees. Extend your arms straight out in front of you and allow your forehead to rest easily on the mat.

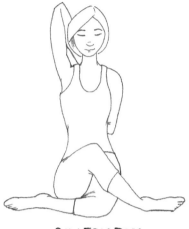

Cow Face Pose

Cow Face Pose

Deep stretch for the hips, ankles, thighs, shoulders, chest, deltoid and triceps. Strengthens back and abdominals

Begin in a seated position. Bend your knees, placing your feet flat on the floor. Bring your left foot under your right knee and place it outside of your right hip. Stack your right knee directly on top of the left, and then move your right foot to the outside of your left hip. Reach your left arm up towards the ceiling with your palm facing forward. Bend your left elbow and drop your left hand to your spine. Reach your right arm to the side with your palm facing down. Rotate your arm so that your palm faces behind you. Bend your right elbow and bring your right hand up the center of your back. Clasp hands if you are able to, otherwise, allow them to stay on your back.

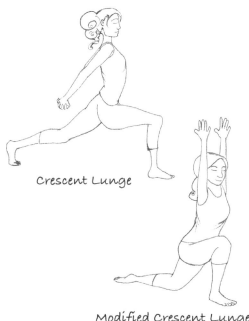

Crescent Lunge

Modified Crescent Lunge

Crescent Lunge (arms up and arms clasps behind back) or modified on back knee

Crescent lunge is a full body pose that increases strength and flexibility.

From downward facing dog, lunge your foot forward into crescent lunge. Your knee and ankle will be straight up and down. Actively pressing back through your back heel, engaging your abdominals, release your shoulders down and back and sink your hips as low as comfortable for you. Your hands can remain on the floor on either side of your front knee, they can be placed on your hips or you can extend your arms up.

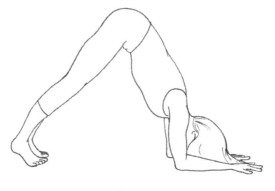

Dolphin Pose

Dolphin

Strengthens the core, arms and legs and an opener for the shoulders

Begin on your hands and knees. Your knees are below your hips and move to your forearms on the floor with your shoulders directly above your wrists. Clasp your palms together and move your forearms to the floor. Curl your toes under and lift your buttocks to the ceiling. Press your ribcage back towards your quads.

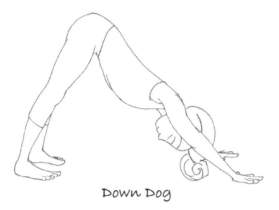

Down Dog

Downward Facing Dog

Stretches the muscles of the back. Releases tension in the shoulders. Stretches and lengthens the hamstrings. Stretches and increases flexibility in the Achilles tendons

Beginning in a modified plank, spread your fingers wide, curl your toes under and press your booty towards the ceiling. Downward facing dog is a resting pose but often does not feel like that we you first begin your yoga practice. After you lift your body into down dog, actively press your rib cage back towards your quads. This decreases the angle at your wrists and makes the pose more comfortable.

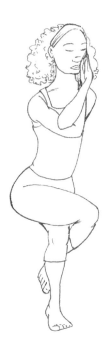

Eagle Pose

Eagle (leg wrapped or tracking beside calf or ankle crossed)

Strengthens and stretches the Achilles and calves. Improves concentration and balance. Stretches the thighs, hips, shoulders and back

Begin in mountain pose. Shift your weight to one leg, bend it, cross the other leg over – the foot of the top leg can track beside the calf or wrap behind the calf. The arms wrap and the hands press together.

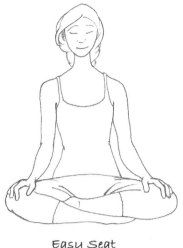

Easy Seat

Easy Seat
Easy Seat forward fold

Sit on the floor. Cross your shins, widen your knees, and slip each foot beneath the opposite knee as you bend your knees and fold the legs in toward your torso. To add the forward fold – hinge from the hips and gently allow your torso to drop forward.

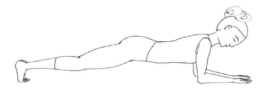

Forearm Plank

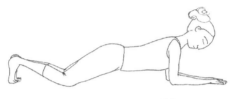

Forearm Plank Modified

Forearm Plank, full and modified

Strengthens the abdominals, biceps, shoulders, triceps back and legs. Increases stamina. Helps with concentration.

From Dolphin – your elbows should be directly under your shoulders and your body in a low plamk position. Lift your belly towards your spine. You will use your core power and your legs to hold you into this position.

Note: you will keep your shoulders pulled down and back and you will tilt your pelvis slightly under to help stabilize your body.

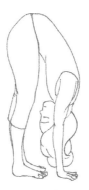

Forward Fold

Forward Fold (arms to floor or holding elbows for ragdoll)

Lengthens the spine. Reduces lower back pain. Increases circulation and lessens fatigue. Alleviates tight hamstrings. It has the benefits of an inversion and stretches the back of the legs, buttocks and back.

Stand with your weight equally distributed between both feet and your feet are about hip width apart. Be aware of how your feel as you slowly fold your body forward. Keep your knees bent initially and engage your belly.

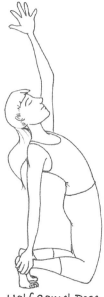

Half Camel Pose

Half Camel Pose

Stretches the entire front of the body, the ankles, thighs and groin and the hip flexors. Strengthens the back muscles and improves the posture

Kneel on the floor with your knees hip width apart. Shins and the tops of the feet are flat on the floor unless you need to curl your toes under to raise your heels higher. For a half camel you will reach one arm back to your heel. In a full camel both hands reach to the heels. Hips stay above the knees. There is a tendency in this pose to allow the hips to drop back towards the feet, maintain the proper alignment.

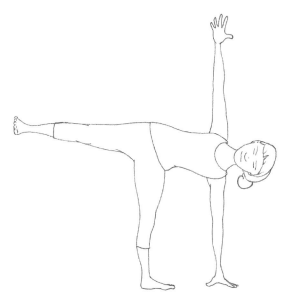

Half Moon Pose

Half Moon Pose

Strengthens the core, ankles, thighs and buttocks. Stretches the groin, hamstrings and calves, shoulders, chest and back

Starting at the front of your mat, move into a low lunge. Place both of your hands on the floor on the outsides of your feet. From here, engage your core, bring your right hand to up towards the ceiling as you rotate your right hip up. The right leg is parallel to the floor with the foot flexed.

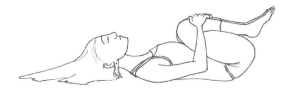

Knees to Chest Pose

Knees to chest

Stretch for the back and groin muscles as it calms for the mind.

Begin on your back and gently pull your knees to your chest. If you need more space, legs can be separated. Relax your shoulders and neck and focus on releasing the back, hips and buttocks.

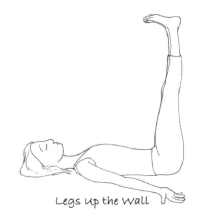

Legs up the Wall

Legs up the wall pose

Usually considered to be a restorative pose at the end of your practice. Many teachers believe that this pose is good for most everything that ails you, including: anxiety, digestive issues, headaches and insomnia.

Lie on your back with your buttock up against the wall and your legs on the wall.

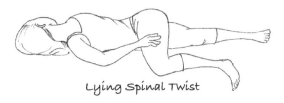

Lying Spinal Twist

Lying Spinal Twist

Stretches and encourages the release of tightness in the back. Stretches the hips, chest, shoulders and upper back

Start by lying on your back, legs straight out. Pull your right knee in to your chest, drop the right knee/leg to the left side and look right. Arms are out in a T.

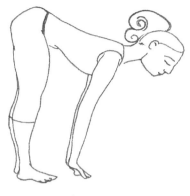

Monkey Pose

Monkey (Standing Half Forward Bend)

Strengthens the back and abdominals.

From a forward fold, engage your belly, lengthen and elongate your back, allow your fingers to reach towards the floor.

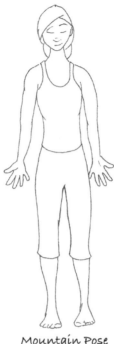

Mountain Pose

Mountain Pose (hands at sides, palms front or reaching to the sky)

Mountain pose is an active pose that is the foundation for all standing poses. You can check your alignment in this pose with your back against the wall. Stand with your heels, sacrum and shoulder blades (but not your head) against the wall.

Provides proper alignment for other standing poses. Restores balance to the body and the mind

Standing in a comfortable stance with your quads engaged, your toes spread; your arms down at our sides, your neck elongated, and your shoulders are relaxed and retracted down.

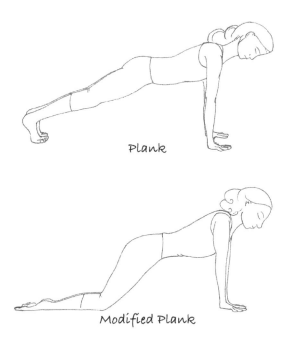

Plank

Modified Plank

Plank, full and modified

Strengthens the abdominals, biceps, shoulders, triceps back and legs. Increases stamina. Helps with concentration.

From Downward facing dog or modified plank or even a forward fold – your hands should be directly under your shoulders and your body in a high pushup position. Lift your belly towards your spine. You will use your core power and your legs to hold you into this position.

Note: you will keep your shoulders pulled down and back and you will tilt your pelvis slightly under to help stabilize your body when in plank.

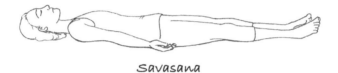

Savasana

Savasana, final relaxation

Relaxes the body and the mind. This is a place where you are take the time to be still. Try to still your body and your mind. If you notice stressful thoughts creeping in, acknowledge them but try to return your focus to your breath.

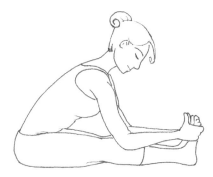

Seated Forward Fold

Seated Forward Fold

Stretches the spine, shoulders and hamstrings, Calms the mind and relieves stress.

Start seated with your legs out in front of you. Hinging at your hips, drop your ribcage towards your thighs. Maintain alignment in your back and only move forward until you feel a stretch in your back and hamstrings. Do not lose your alignment as you move forward.

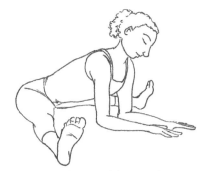

Seated Straddle Fold

Seated Straddle Fold

Stretches the inside and back of legs. Strengthens the core.

Sit on the floor with your legs as wide apart as you are comfortable. Hinging at your hips, drop your ribcage towards the floor. Maintain alignment in your back and only move forward until you feel a stretch in your back and hamstrings. Do not lose your alignment as you move forward.

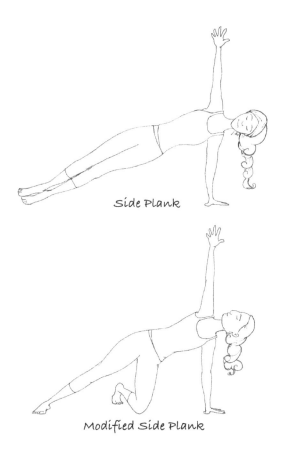

Side Plank

Modified Side Plank

Side Plank, full and modified

Strengthens the arms, core and legs. Stretches and strengthens the wrists. Improves balance.

Begin in downward facing dog. Lower your body into plank pose. Step your feet together, press your weight through your right hand, roll your body to the right, balancing on the outer edge of your right foot. Stack your left foot on top of your right foot and keep your legs straight. Extend your left arm to the ceiling. Remember to keep your core engaged and if you need more support, you can drop a knee or separate your feet.

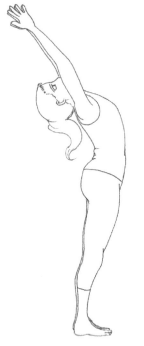

Standing Backbend

Standing Backbend

Strengthens your back and a modification for wheel pose.

Beginning in mountain pose, lift your right arm up to the ceiling and your left arm down your left thigh. Lifting from your chest and ribcage, reach your chest to the sky. This is a gentle backbend and can be used as a warmup for more intense backbends. It can also be a standalone pose.

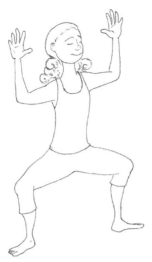

Sun God Pose

Sun God

Opens your hips and strengthens your legs. This is an energizing and grounding pose.

Begin in a standing position with your feet approximately 36" apart. Everyone is different, adjust the spacing for your body and your flexibility. Bend your knees and keep the knees and ankles in alignment and keep your knees pressing back.

Yoga for Strength
Sun Salute A

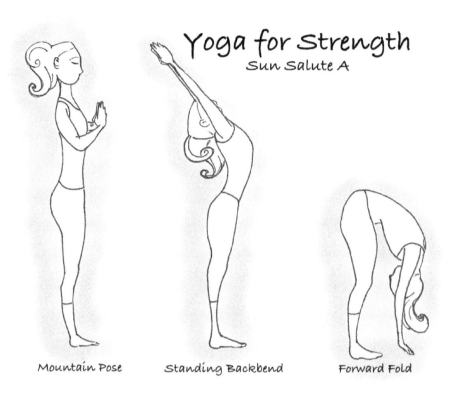

Mountain Pose   Standing Backbend   Forward Fold

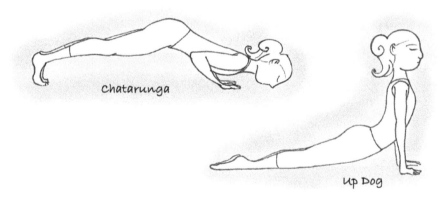

Chatarunga

Up Dog

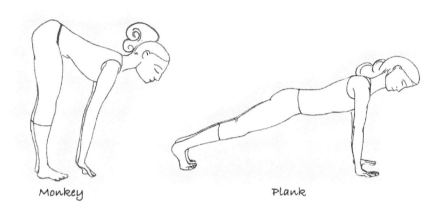

Monkey

Plank

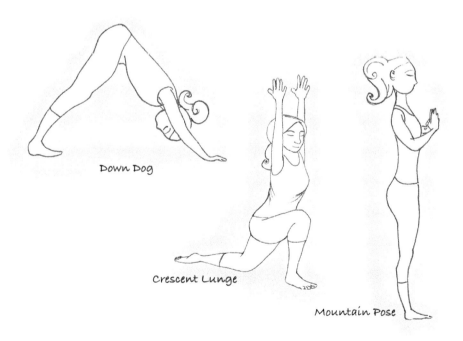

Down Dog

Crescent Lunge

Mountain Pose

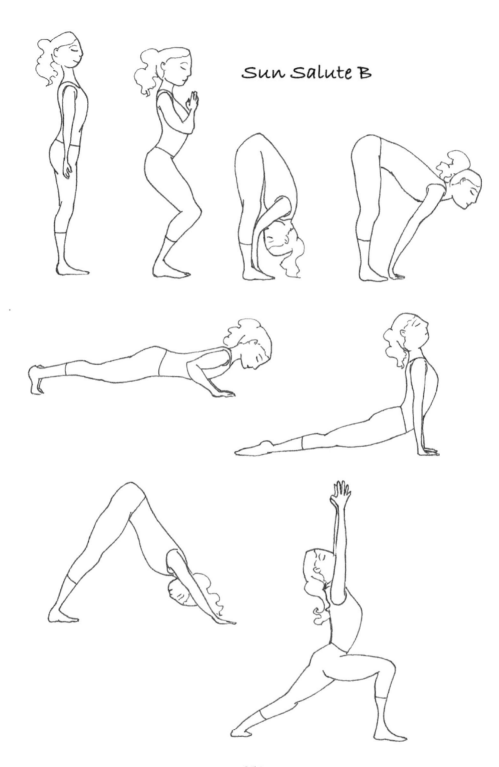

Sun Salute B

Yoga Practice Notes

Yoga for Courage

Sun Salute C

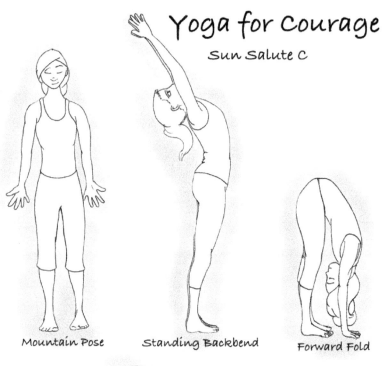

Mountain Pose   Standing Backbend   Forward Fold

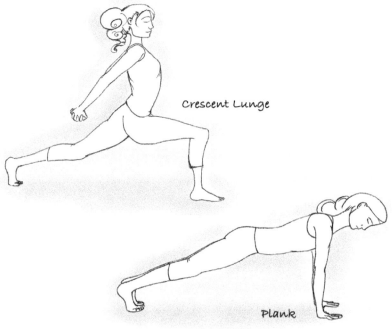

Crescent Lunge

Plank

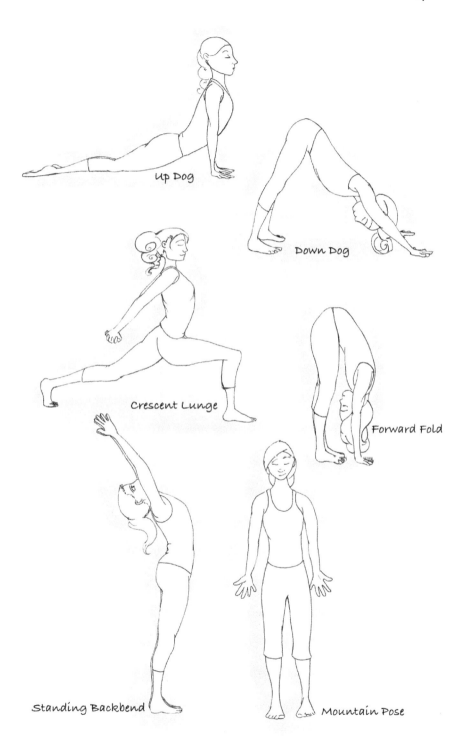

Up Dog

Down Dog

Crescent Lunge

Forward Fold

Standing Backbend

Mountain Pose

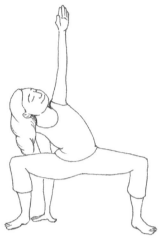

Temple Pose

Temple Pose

Hip opening pose. Strengthens thighs and waist and an overall core strengthener.

Begin in Sun God pose. Maintaining lower body alignment, reach your right arm straight down towards the floor behind your right leg as the left arm reaches up to the ceiling. Repeat other side.

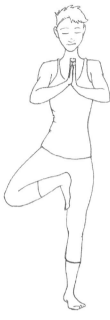

Tree Pose

Tree Pose

Improves the posture and elongates the spine. Strengthens the knees and ankles. Stretches the groin muscles and helps with balance and focus.

Begin in Mountain Pose, extend and lengthen your spine. Do not let your body weight drop into the hip of the leg you are standing on.

Move the sole of your right foot onto your calf or inner thigh. The only place we do not want our foot is on our knee. Keep your hips even and aligned with each other.

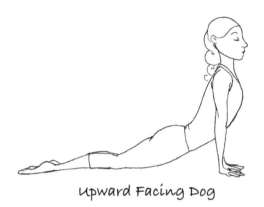

Upward Facing Dog

Upward Facing Dog

Stretches the entire front of your torso as it strengthens the muscles in your arms, shoulders and back.

Press palms and tops of feet into the mat. You will use your quadriceps, booty and abdominals to help lift your thighs off the mat. Your chest and torso will be slightly in front of your hands and your torso will hang between your arms.

Note: relax your shoulders down and back.

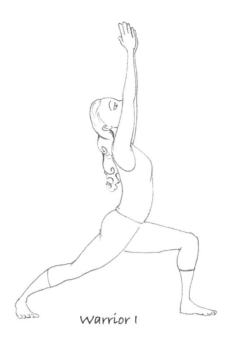

Warrior I

Warrior I

Strengthens the feet, ankles, knees and legs. Helps to relieve stiffness in the back, shoulders and neck. Prepares the body for backbends later in your practice.

From downward facing dog, lunge your left leg forward between your hands and bend the front knee to a 90 degree angle. Set your back foot flat and out at a 45-60 degree angle. Press into the outer edge of your back foot. Square your pelvis and shoulders to the front of your mat.

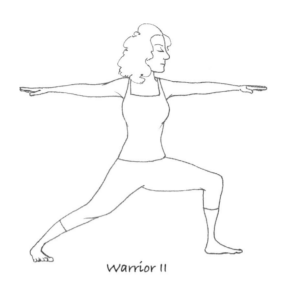

Warrior II

Warrior II

Strengthens the feet, ankles, knees and legs. Opens and stretches the hips. Increases endurance and stamina.

From downward facing dog, lunge your left leg forward between your hands and bend the front knee to a 90 degree angle. Set your back foot flat and out at a 45-60 degree angle. Press into the outer edge of your back foot. Square your pelvis and shoulders to the side of your mat. Extend your arms out firmly away from the midline of your body. Look out over your front hand.

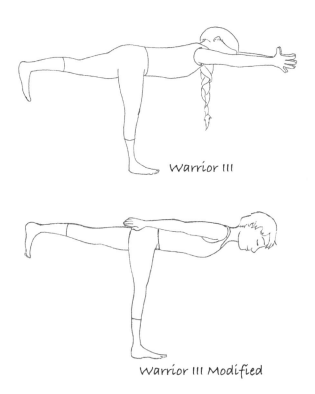

Warrior III

Warrior III Modified

Warrior III (with balancing stick and airplane modifications)

Strengthens the core and glutes. Stretches the hamstrings. A challenging balance pose, as well as an endurance pose.

Standing in Mountain Pose extend arms overhead or down at your sides. Extend one leg behind you as you balance on the other. Hinge from your hips and lower your upper body until leg and upper body are parallel. Lengthen in opposite directions away from the midline of your body. Arms at your side for balancing stick. Breathe. Repeat on other leg.

About the Author

A born educator and compassionate healer, Cathleen Kahn teaches people to see physical fitness as a path to positive change in their lives. Working as a yogi, wellness expert, and the founder and co-owner of CatFit Yoga, she helps her clients find sustainable paths to health, happiness, and self-love.

She's always loved yoga, but it wasn't until Cathleen survived a battle with breast cancer that it became central to her life. She says, "After cancer, I lived yoga. When I lost my hair, yoga didn't care how I looked. When I felt betrayed by my body, the yoga mat welcomed me. Yoga was therapeutic and a place of acceptance and healing for me during and after my diagnosis."

When she's not teaching, writing, or speaking, Cathleen loves to travel, volunteer, and savor a great glass of red wine. She enjoys learning as much as teaching and strives to make a lasting and positive difference in the lives of everyone she meets.

CPSIA information can be obtained
at www.ICGtesting.com
Printed in the USA
LVHW090423171218
600716LV00002B/352/P